double take | the story of twins

double take | the story of twins

Daniel Jussim

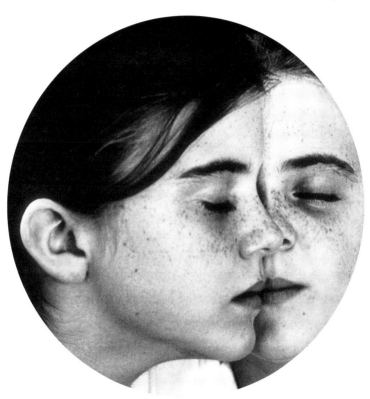

viking

VIKING
Published by the Penguin Group
Penguin Putnam Books for Young Readers, 345 Hudson Street,
New York, New York 10014, U.S.A.
Penguin Books Ltd, 27 Wrights Lane, London W8 5TZ, England
Penguin Books Australia Ltd, Ringwood, Victoria, Australia
Penguin Books Canada Ltd, 10 Alcorn Avenue, Toronto, Ontario,
Canada M4V 3B2
Penguin Books (N.Z.) Ltd, 182-190 Wairau Road, Auckland 10,
New Zealand

Penguin Books Ltd, Registered Offices: Harmondsworth,
Middlesex, England

First published in 2001 by Viking,
a division of Penguin Putnam Books for Young Readers.
1 2 3 4 5 6 7 8 9 10

Front jacket photo and title page: © David Teplica, MD, MFA, courtesy of the Collected Image, Evanston, Ill.; pages viii, 1, 17 and 18: courtesy of Lisa and Jennifer Gould; page 2: © G. Shih and R. Kessel/Visuals Unlimited; pages 4 and 11: courtesy of Andrea Messina; page 7: courtesy of Erin Moriarty; page 8: © Wildlife Conservation Society, headquartered at the Bronx Zoo; pages 10, 12, and back jacket: photos by Daniel Jussim; pages 14 and 15: Kiefel Photography, photos by Darcy Kiefel; pages 19 and 20: courtesy of Kathy Martin; page 22: Imogen Cunningham Trust, photo by Imogen Cunningham, copyright © 1978; page 25: Imogen Cunningham Trust, photo by Ron Partridge, copyright © 1999; pages 26, 31, 43, 52, 53: AP/Wide World Photos; page 32: courtesy of Dr. Nancy L. Segal, author of *Entwined Lives: Twins and What They Tell Us About Human Behavior*; page 34: AP by Tony Dejak, copyright © 1993; page 35: copyright © 1998 by David Fields, reprinted with permission from *Twins*, text by Ruth and Rachel Sandweiss, photos by David Fields, published by Running Press, Philadelphia and London; page 37: Disabled Sports Marketing; page 44: courtesy of *The Tampa Tribune*; page 47: Corbis Sygma, photo by Dana Fineman copyright © 1999; page 49: Corbis Sygma; pages 55 and 66: photos by Steve Wewerka, Impact Visuals; pages 58, 59, 61, 62, 63: courtesy of the Mütter Museum, Philadelphia, Pa.; page 68: courtesy of the Los Angeles Music Awards and Al Bowen.

The photo that appears on the jacket is called *Monozygotic Fusion* and was taken by Dr. David Teplica in 1988. Dr. Teplica, a plastic surgeon in Chicago, has photographed over six thousand twin portraits since 1988.

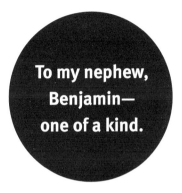

To my nephew,
Benjamin—
one of a kind.

Thanks to my editor, Jill Davis, and to the following people for their generous help in research and editing: Susan Alt, Catherine Frank, Elizabeth Goldleaf, Genevieve Goldleaf, Gillian Martin, Janet Pascal, Nancy Segal, Devan Sipher, Glenn Slater, and Wendy Wilf. I am also grateful to the people who agreed to be interviewed for "Five Dynamic Duos," and to those who provided photographs. Finally, special thanks to Stacey Luftig for her love, encouragement, and keen editorial eye.

contents

1 the world of twins

10 five dynamic duos

26 separated at birth

34 more amazing stories

43 multiples

55 conjoined twins

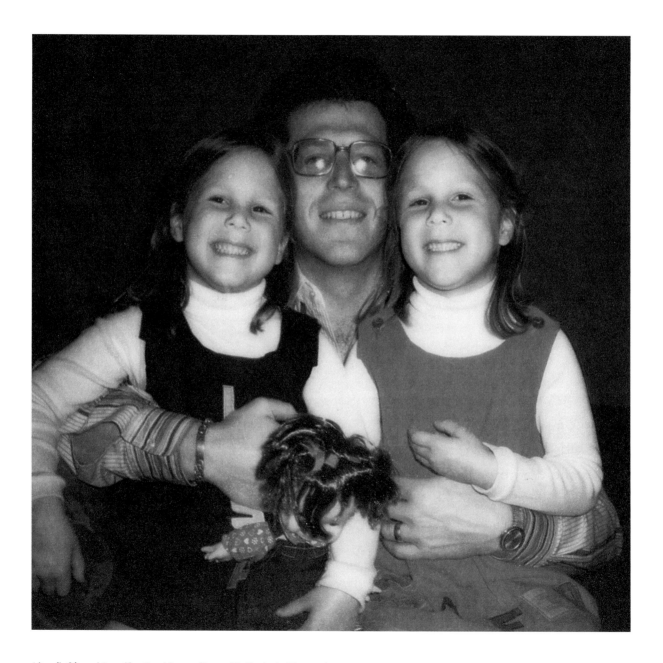

Lisa (left) and Jennifer Gould, age five, with their dad in 1976

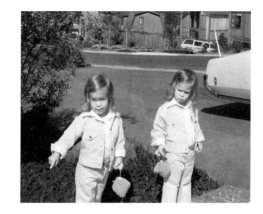

the world of twins

On the playground at their school, two girls in first grade chatted away, totally absorbed in each other's company. A classmate approached, staring at them. "Why don't you two switch places a few times," she suggested, "while I close my eyes and spin around. Then I'll try to guess who is who."

The girls looked at their classmate with disdain. "We're not in a zoo!" they declared. Then, as one, they turned and stormed off.

It was just another day in the lives of identical twins Lisa and Jennifer Gould. Sure, they worked together, played together, shared wardrobes, and looked as alike as peas in a pod, but that didn't mean they liked being compared.

It's hard, though, to resist being fascinated by twins and comparing them. They're the same, yet they're different. As we'll see in the next chapter, Jennifer and Lisa are grown up now; they have a great deal in common, and are very involved in each other's life. Sometimes

ABOVE: Jennifer (left) and Lisa in 1974, age three

they catch themselves making their own comparisons. Watching Lisa train for running a marathon, Jennifer aches to join her. She knows a bad knee won't let her cover such long distances, but somewhere in the back of her mind is a voice saying, *We're twins—I can do anything she does.*

Twins have something that most people want—they grow up with constant companionship, so they're hardly ever lonely. They have a soul mate who understands them when no one else can. But they face unique challenges also. For while the world—always comparing— sees a single pair, twins are two, too. They must develop a sense of themselves as individuals. They must understand that their tastes and talents, whether running marathons or playing piano, won't always be shared.

• HOW TWINS ARE MADE •

Human conception occurs inside a woman's uterus when a sperm cell from the father fertilizes an egg cell from the mother. The fertilized egg, or zygote, then attaches to the wall of the uterus and develops into an embryo and then a fetus. In most births one baby, a "singleton," is born about nine months later. With twins, however, there is a twist, and two children are born. How does this happen?

Twins can be identical or fraternal. Like singletons, identical twins develop from a single fertilized egg. But early in the zygote's development, it splits and

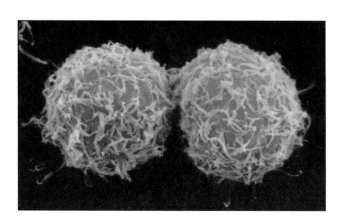

After being fertilized, a human egg cell splits, creating twins.

two embryos are formed. These grow into two babies who have the same genes (see box), and are thus genetically identical. Both babies will be boys, or both girls; identical twins always share the same sex.

Fraternal twins occur twice as often as identical twins. They develop when two eggs in the uterus are fertilized by two sperm. This creates two zygotes, which eventually become two babies who are not genetically identical. On average, they share half of the same genes— just like any other pair of siblings. Fraternals may be both boys, both girls, or, unlike identicals, a boy-girl pair.

Fraternal-twin births run in families, but identical-twin births seem to occur randomly. Let's say, for instance, that your mother were a fraternal twin. There would be a higher

GENES AND WHAT THEY MEAN

Genes are instructions that tell the body how to do its job. These instructions are recorded in every cell of our bodies. A baby's genes come from its mother and father. Genes give people their appearance. Because of genes, a person looks like a person, not a dog or a goldfish. (Plants and animals have genes too. They make a cat look like a cat, not an iguana.) Genes make someone short or tall, blond or brunet, blue eyed or green eyed or brown eyed. Everyone is special, and no two people look exactly alike. But most children look at least a bit like their biological parents, and that's because of genes too. Identical twins share the same genes, and that's why their appearance is usually so similar. And because genes can affect behavior and personality too, these twins may share habits and talents.

4

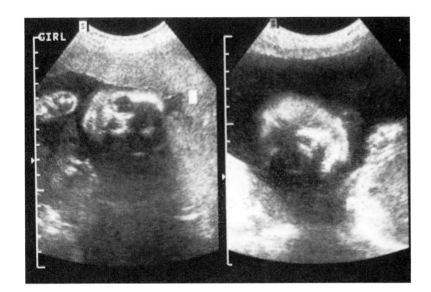

A split-screen sonogram showing twins in their mother's uterus at 22 weeks. You'll meet these twins—Josie and Benjy—in the next chapter. (The word GIRL in the upper left-hand corner refers to Josie.)

chance that if you became a parent, you would have fraternal twins yourself. But if, instead, she were an identical twin, your chances of parenting identicals would be unchanged.

While only identicals are a genetic match, all twins are "wombmates"—they develop together in the uterus, sharing that tight space until they are born. Some scientists believe that they compete for resources—such as space and blood flow from the mother—from early in the pregnancy. They also may develop some kind of emotional relationship. Sonograms, which let doctors see inside the uterus, have shown twins kissing, stroking, and punching each other.

Although most twins are born minutes apart, sometimes a long gap separates their entrance into the world. For instance, on August 13, 1980, twenty-one-year-old Terri Plompen of Algoma, Wisconsin, gave birth to a daughter named Robyn Theresa, but Robyn Theresa's twin didn't appear that day. It wasn't until four weeks later that her sister, Renee Marle, was born, setting a record for the longest time period between births in Wisconsin.

Sometimes nature goes one step beyond twins, and triplets (three babies born at once), quadruplets (four babies), or even more develop. These "supertwins" may be identical or fraternal. They may even be a combination of both. This could occur, for example, if two eggs were fertilized by two sperm to form two zygotes, and then one of the zygotes split. The split zygotes would become identical twins; the other zygote would be their fraternal triplet.

Finally, a rarer type of twinning may occur when a zygote splits, but after an unusual delay. Conjoined twins—genetically identical and physically connected—may develop. Often these twins are joined at the chest or the side.

• THE TWIN BOOM •

If you know a twin or are one, there is a good reason—more twins and multiples are being born now than ever before. Consider these U.S. statistics:

- Today about 1 in 36 births is a twin birth.
- In 1998, 110,670 pairs of twins were born, which represented a 62 percent increase over the number of twin births in 1980.
- In 1998 the number of multiple births—triplets or more—reached 7,625. In 1980, by contrast, there were 1,337 such births.

Why is this happening? Two reasons: First, women are having babies at a later age than they used to. When they get pregnant between ages thirty-five and forty, they are more likely to have twins, because they produce more of a certain hormone. This hormone encourages the release of eggs into the uterus, making fraternal twins a greater possibility.

The other reason is that more couples are resorting to fertility treatments when they find it difficult to conceive. These treatments—fertility drugs and in-vitro fertilization—make it more likely that women will produce more than one egg, in turn increasing the odds of having fraternal twins. While having babies later in life and/or using fertility treatments increases the chances of giving birth to fraternal twins, the odds of having identical twins remains unaffected.

• THE MEANING OF "IDENTICAL" •

When it comes to twins, identical does not mean "looking exactly alike." Rather, it means "sharing the same genes." While most identical twins bear a striking resemblance to each other and have many qualities in common, others may have significant differences. This is because of the influence of the environment—and "environment" includes the womb that was home before birth. The different positions of twin fetuses in the uterus and their abilities to get nutrients there can affect them later in life.

Twins Kelley and Missi Seemuth were identical but looked very different. Their different appearance resulted from Kelley being deprived of oxygen and nutrition when she was a fetus. When they were born, Kelley weighed 1 pound 14 ounces less than Missi. Kelley was right-handed and Missi was left-handed. At eight years old, Kelley was 5 inches shorter and 9 pounds lighter than her sister.

On the other hand, it is possible for twins who are actually fraternal to *appear* identical. Though fraternals come from two zygotes, they can, by chance, inherit many of the same genes. This can happen with any pair of siblings, even nontwins.

Because fraternals may have a close resemblance, and identicals may not, it is easy for doctors and parents to make mistakes when typing twins. Many identical twins do not think they look alike, and many twins of both types are unsure of their status.

Take the case of Erin Moriarty and her twin sister, Sheelah. Erin, a correspondent for the CBS news program *48 Hours*, and Sheelah, an airline executive, were told all their lives that

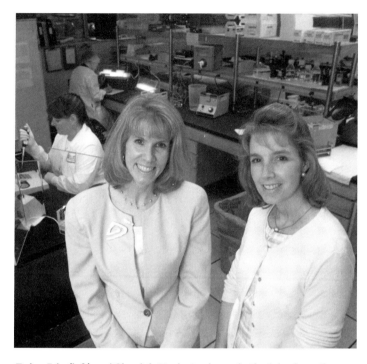

Twins Erin (left) and Sheelah Moriarty shown in the lab where they learned that they were fraternal, not identical, twins

they were identical. That's what the doctor who delivered them said, and what their mother believed. Sheelah acknowledged that she always seemed a bit taller when they were growing up, but insisted they were identical: "It's been my truth all my life, that's what I've been told and so I had no reason to question it."

But Erin was more skeptical. She thought they were fraternal "because my sister tans better, she has smoother hair than I do and she looks different than I do."

The only way to know for sure about twin type is to get a DNA test. In identical twins, DNA, the substance that makes up our genes, is exactly the same; in fraternal twins it is not. Erin and Sheelah went to a laboratory, where they gave tissue samples by rubbing a swab against the inside of their cheeks. A geneticist then compared the DNA in this tissue. Because only half of the six genetic "markers" on their DNA matched, the geneticist concluded that the two were in fact fraternal twins. A stunned Sheelah asked the geneticist, "And we're saying this test is accurate? There's no question?" Erin's reaction? She turned to Sheelah and said, "*You* have to tell mom."

Doctors believe that it is important for twins to know if they're identical. It's not just a

7

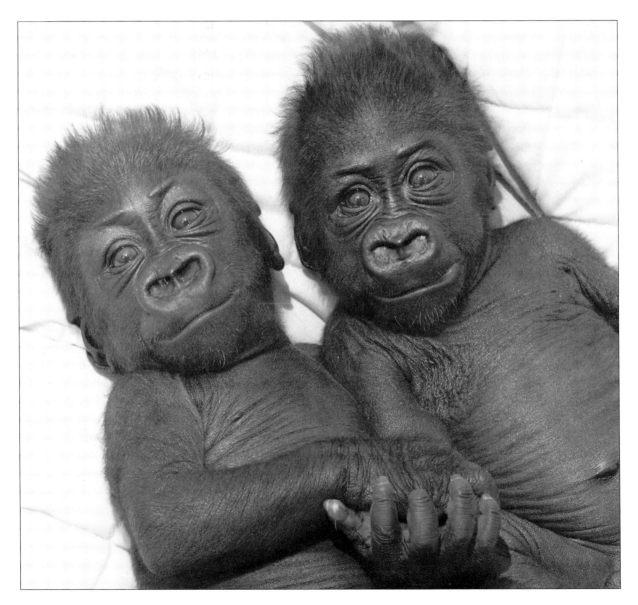

Fraternal male twin gorillas Ngoma and Tambo at two months of age. They were born in August 1994 at the Bronx Zoo.

matter of curiosity. Genes can influence whether we get certain diseases, so when someone gets a disease his identical twin may be at high risk of contracting the same illness. A fraternal twin would be at lower risk. If doctors know the twin type, they can take the correct measures.

• ANIMAL TWINS •

Twinning doesn't occur just among people, but happens in the nonhuman animal world too. Cows and bulls produce fraternal twins in one out of fifty births. Horses produce twins also, and as you may know if you have a pet, dogs and cats are usually born in litters (the name of multiple births in animals). An animal known as the nine-banded armadillo has a unique talent—it almost always produces identical quadruplets.

Primates, such as chimpanzees and gorillas, sometimes give birth to twins too, although rarely in captivity. That may explain the fuss made over the birth of twin gorillas Ngoma and Tambo in August 1994 at the Bronx Zoo in New York City. These fraternal male twins, who come from an endangered species known as the Western lowland gorilla, had such similar appearances that their caretakers thought they must be identical. However, DNA tests proved them to be fraternal twins. Their faces are extremely similar in the photo, taken in their infancy. Even three years after the gorillas' birth, people working with them had to rely on small differences in the shapes of their heads and their nostrils to distinguish them.

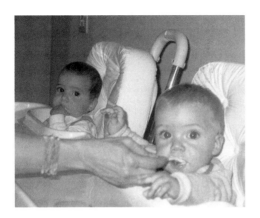

five dynamic duos

In this chapter, we'll profile five sets of twins—identical, fraternal, same sex, different sex, young, old—with a wide range of experiences and outlooks. Being a twin has different consequences for different people, but certain themes run through many of these twins' lives: the joy of having a friend from birth; the problems and pleasures of looking strikingly like someone else; the unusual family relationships; the complex social dynamics. Whether you're a twin or not, you'll be fascinated by how these pairs deal with each other and the rest of the world.

• JOSIE AND BENJY: WIGGLING WITH DELIGHT •

Andrea Messina had given birth before—to her son, Teddy—so she knew what it was like to carry a baby. And she knew that this time it felt different. Three months into her pregnancy, she felt an unfamiliar, heavy weight in her belly when she bent over to wash her face. Glancing in the mirror, Andrea thought she looked four months pregnant, not three.

ABOVE: Josie (left) and Benjy, age seven months

By four months, she had gained nine pounds. Was it twins? She didn't want to believe it. Two newborns would need so much attention. And Teddy was still just two years old.

But she had an additional concern. Her baby's weight felt odd to her, and she started to fear it was dead. She went to see her midwife, a person who helps women with childbirth in place of a doctor.

The midwife listened to Andrea's belly through a stethoscope attached to a small speaker, allowing Andrea to listen too. The rhythmic sound Andrea heard was music to her ears: the strong heartbeat of a baby. Then the midwife moved the stethoscope a bit. As if in a dream, Andrea heard a telltale thumping and the midwife's exclamation: "There's another heartbeat!"

"I almost died," Andrea says. "I covered my face. I was speechless." An examination done with an ultrasound machine a few days later gave Andrea a view of her twins moving around inside her uterus.

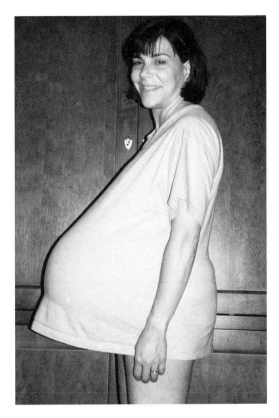

Andrea Messina shown the evening before giving birth to Josie and Benjy

Andrea became tremendous, adding more than sixty pounds to her thin, 5 foot 2 ½ inch frame over the pregnancy. At seven months, she couldn't sit in restaurants where the tables and chairs were immovable, because she couldn't fit. She couldn't walk more than four blocks at a time, or carry anything heavy.

One day when she was out with Teddy, he suddenly ran toward the street. Andrea chased him, but couldn't keep up. He stopped in time, but Andrea, in pain, realized she could no longer run. Frighteningly, she'd have to rely on two-and-a-half-year-old Teddy not to misbehave this way again.

At eight months, unable to balance herself properly, Andrea would trip over her feet and go down like a tree—right on her ballooned belly. She worried the babies would be hurt. She also worried about herself.

Finally, Josephine and Benjamin were born at 39 weeks by cesarean section (most twins come out sooner). Andrea hired a twins expert to show her how to pick up one baby when she had the other one in her arms. To breast-feed her babies at the same time, Andrea had to buy a special U-shaped pillow that slanted in to keep the babies to her breast. Andrea and husband John also had to buy more baby clothes and started purchasing formula and diapers in bulk.

In the beginning, when Andrea lived in Brooklyn, New York, she faced the challenge of getting her babies into the subway. Many times strangers helped her, but once a passerby looked at Andrea struggling alone to carry them, exclaimed, "That's amazing!" and walked

12

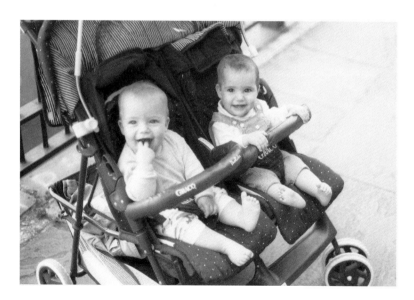

Benjy (left) and Josie in their double stroller

on without lifting a finger. Eventually Andrea and John moved their clan into a house in New Jersey and bought a minivan.

The twins' personalities are different. According to her mom, Josie is alert, expressive, and looks wise beyond her years. Benjy is good natured, smiles at everybody, and expects to be happy. When he sees you, his eyes light up, as though he were thinking, *You're going to make me laugh, aren't you?* Josie, on the other hand, looks at you with suspicion. She's more sensitive and wary.

Though caring for them is an enormous challenge, it's been a little easier than Andrea had thought it would be. The pair are a source of endless pleasure—even for Teddy. Though he got jealous at first, he is now proud to be big brother to twins. And the feeling is mutual. One of Josie's first words was "Teddy." "They light up when Teddy comes near," Andrea says. Teddy will sing a song or make faces and watch the twins "wiggle with delight."

• MAX AND ANDY: PUSHING THEIR LIMITS •

In 1991, two three-year-old identical twin brothers were living in a big farmhouse in Russia. The farmhouse, located in a town outside of Moscow, was used as a group home for disabled orphans. Before these twins were born, they were injured in their mother's uterus. The umbilical cord, which provides nutrients to the fetus, became wrapped around their legs and cut off blood circulation. As a result, the brothers were born with gangrene in their legs, and needed operations to remove the infected limbs. One boy had both legs amputated about five inches below the knee, the other had one leg amputated six inches below the hip. Unfortunately, doctors could not fit them with artificial legs that would let them walk well. So, playing in the orphanage, one of the twins walked around on his knees, and the other hopped around on his one good leg.

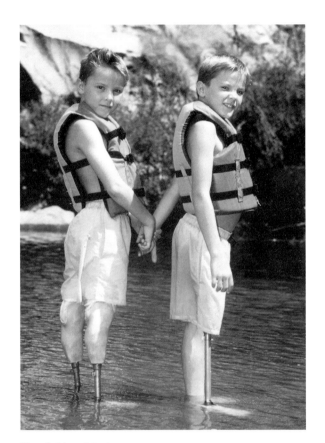

Max (left) and Andy

One day in December of that year, an Illinois man was reading a newspaper article about the plight of Russian orphans. The article discussed the disabled twins. This man had lost a leg himself, as a soldier in the Vietnam War. As he read, something struck him. *I could do something for these boys that someone with two good legs could not—because I experience what they experience.*

He decided to adopt the twins. The press was so intrigued by the story that upon returning to the United States, the man, Ron Greenfield, and the twins, Max and Andy, were greeted at the airport by about thirty photographers and reporters. But Ron knew that the most important thing was the twins' health. He got them to a good hospital, where the boys could be looked at and fitted with prostheses, devices that would let them walk.

They were thrilled when they could stand up and walk normally for the first time, but in addition to learning this new skill, the boys had to learn a new language—English. They are now eleven, their English is perfect, and with their high-tech prostheses—made of metal and fiberglass, with an artificial foot made of carbon fiber—they play basketball together, ride bikes, and even swim. "I can pretty much do what I want with these legs," declares Max.

"I push them," Ron says. "I don't let them use their artificial legs as an excuse for not being able to do something." And Ron, who is raising Max and Andy with his wife, Debbie, is a natural role model, showing his kids all the possibilities. He wears shorts—"I don't hide my artificial leg"—and wears out his own prostheses water skiing, snow skiing, and playing baseball and volleyball. He's also in a unique position to help his children with their equipment—if one of his kids has a pain, he knows from the type of hurt that Max or Andy doesn't have his artificial leg on right. He can tell his son that he's got it twisted or there is air in the bottom.

Ron, Max, and Andy get some curious looks from strangers when they are out together. According to Ron, a common question they get is, "Gosh, were you guys all in an accident?"

And the brothers have encountered some nastiness: "Some kids will just walk away from me and tell their friends all about my leg and start making fun of me," says Max. But they have found ways to deal with the challenge. Andy says when he meets new kids, "I talk to them first and tell them what happened. Then they just ignore it and talk to me like a normal kid."

The two have few memories of the orphanage where they started life—just the Russian words *da*, for "yes," and *nyet*, meaning "no."

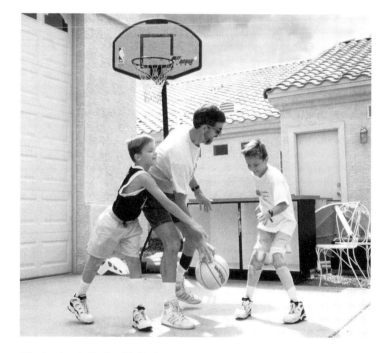

Playing basketball with Dad

15

Max says that he only had soup and bread for lunch and dinner. But that has all changed. Now Andy's favorite meal is "two chicken legs and corn on the cob and refried beans and mashed potatoes and lettuce."

• LISA AND JENNIFER: SEPARATION ANXIETY •

When Jennifer Gould was a child, she had a recurring dream in which a masked person would come in and kill her parents and her little sister. Only when he was about to kill Lisa, her identical twin, would Jennifer scream and wake herself up. Jennifer still has a special dread of Lisa dying. It makes her nervous when her sister flies. "It's my biggest fear—losing her," she says.

Jennifer is at her happiest when she's with her sister. The feeling goes back to when they were growing up near San Francisco and the two were inseparable. They shared wardrobes, and when they were ten years old, they started collecting pennies together to save for a wedding dress. They planned to buy it many years in the future for whoever got married first. Later, the other would have her turn to wear it.

The twins also played folk music together—Lisa strumming a guitar and singing, Jennifer playing drums and singing harmony. They came to each other's rescue: Lisa, for instance, would help Jennifer type last-minute school papers at three in the morning. And they had fun with their identical appearances, trading places and fooling their boyfriends and teachers.

When it came time to go to college, the sisters ended up together again, both choosing UCLA, both choosing the same sorority, both choosing to share an apartment together their senior year. When they dated, they went out only with those boys who understood and accepted the twins' close bond. They thought no one could come between them.

A few years later, while they were celebrating their twenty-sixth birthday, this belief was put to a test. The twins were living in California, but Lisa had a boyfriend in Spain. After the sisters had dinner out, Lisa wanted to share the day with him. But when the couple spoke on the telephone for a half hour, Jennifer got angry, feeling deprived of Lisa's attention—on a day that was special to *them*. The anger didn't last, but something was different . . . and a bigger change was coming.

Lisa will soon be married to the man she telephoned that day, and they will move to Oklahoma—far from Jennifer, who will remain in California, near where she grew up. Though the sisters will probably still talk by phone or by e-mail every day and though they've lived apart before, this time their separation will be more permanent.

Jennifer will miss having someone so close to her to share things with, especially because she has no boyfriend of her own right now.

Lisa feels a little guilty. She's starting a new adventure, which may make the separation easier for her. She imagines Jennifer taking walks alone through the

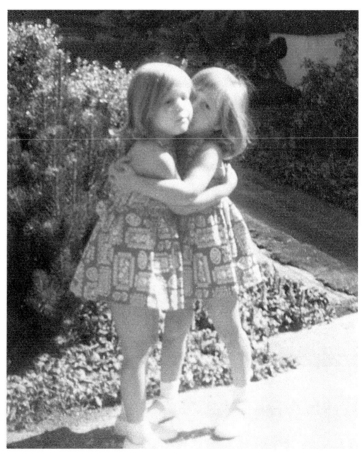

Lisa (left) and Jennifer Gould, age four

places they've always gone to-gether, and it makes her sad.

As for Lisa's fiancé, he and Jennifer get along well. But Lisa says he is sometimes jealous of the sisters, and he fears that if Lisa had to choose between him and Jennifer in a life-or-death situation, she wouldn't save him. Lisa doesn't know what she would do. "It makes me feel horrible. They're such different relationships and such different types of love. In a way my relationship with Jennifer is a lot deeper—we've known each other since before we were born."

Lisa and Jennifer recently took the pennies they'd collected since age ten—16,000 of them—and bought wedding shoes (the dress was too expensive). Lisa is going to wear them first. When the time comes for Jennifer to get married, the shoes will fit her same-size feet.

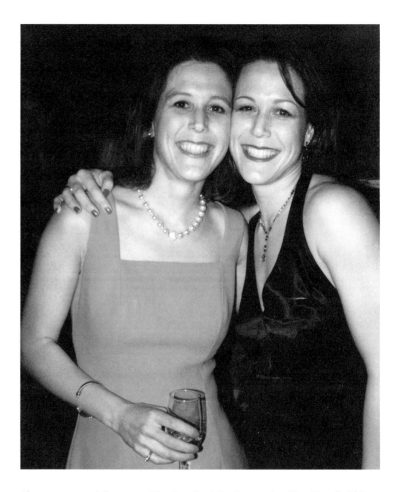

These twenty-eight-year-old twins don't look exactly alike. Lisa (left) has a freckle on her left cheek and Jennifer doesn't, and that's how most people tell them apart. Also, their smiles differ, Jennifer's hair is curlier, and Lisa's eyes are rounder, while Jennifer's are more almond shaped. Of course, a person's appearance is not merely a matter of flesh and bone. The two can also be distinguished by their personalities, which affect the way they carry themselves and the way they talk. "We're animated differently," says Jennifer.

• KATHY AND ARLEEN: A BOND FORMED BY TRAGEDY •

Kathy and Arleen Martin, age sixty, are a good example of how identical twins can be very different—even from the time of their birth. Kathy is healthy, an artist and a former nurse. She married a doctor and had two children. Arleen is mentally disabled and has the intelligence of a five-year-old. She has been cared for by others her whole life. How did the paths of these sisters come to diverge so sharply?

When the twins' mother was pregnant, she told her doctor she thought she felt two babies. The arrogant doctor did not believe her and said, "How would you know? You've never had a child before." However, she went into labor several weeks early, and when she was giving birth the doctor realized he'd made a grave error and exclaimed, "Oh my God, there is another one!"

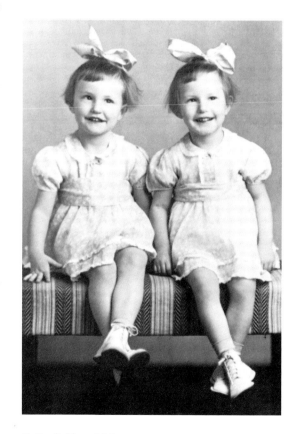

In delivering Kathy, the physician, not expecting a second baby, injured Arleen. As a result of her injury, Arleen began having dramatic seizures at nine months. She was also severely retarded.

Kathy recalls what it was like to grow up in a small town in upstate New York with a twin whose life was dominated by illness. Arleen's terrifying seizures could last all night. They were extremely dangerous because they could cause

Kathy (left) and Arleen, age 5 ½

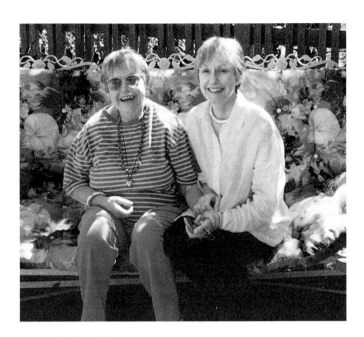

Arleen (left) and Kathy in 1998

further brain damage. In the mid-1940s, doctors could stop this kind of seizure only by anesthetizing Arleen with the chemical ether.

Kathy remembers standing in a hallway at night as a child, watching a doctor sitting on the edge of her sister's bed. "I saw him place a gauze mask over her nose and mouth, watched him drip the ether into this mask."

Kathy has stood by her sister her whole life. As a young child, Kathy made her own friends but included Arleen in their play. She also was a fierce fighter brave enough to hit boys who teased her sister. In high school Kathy saw to it that Arleen was made an honorary member of her sorority. And as an adult, when the twins' mom became ill and could no longer care for Arleen, Kathy took Arleen in to her San Francisco home. She eventually placed her in a nearby group home, where she could get the care she needed.

But in her youth Kathy suffered for having a sick and disabled twin. Because her sister was so ill while her own health was so vigorous, Kathy would seldom get the attention she needed when she wasn't well herself. When Kathy had stomach pains at age seventeen, her mother dismissed her complaints until a doctor said that her appendix was about to burst.

When Kathy started dating at age fifteen, there was a big difference in the twins' appearances. Kathy was tiny, but Arleen had gained an enormous amount of weight because she wasn't active. This embarrassed Kathy, and she would feel insecure about it until boys got to know her sister.

And there was a lot of sorrow to deal with. Kathy attended junior high school with the grandchildren of the doctor who botched the twins' delivery. She says, "I used to look at them and think how healthy looking they were. And think about the fact that their grandfather had devastated my sister's life."

In spite of their differences, the two have things in common. They both have their parents' tough, stubborn, Scottish immigrants' personalities. And their feelings for each other are clear. On a recent outing, on which Kathy took Arleen to physical therapy, to get her hair cut, and then to lunch, Arleen tearfully told Kathy, "I love you."

"In a very deep way," says Kathy, "she understands that we are a pair. And that she would do anything for me and I would do anything for her."

• RON AND PAD: LOOKING FOR TROUBLE •

Twins Ron and Pad Partridge are eighty-three, which means they grew up during the Great Depression. There were few jobs and their family conserved in every way they could. Instead of buying drinking glasses, they took beer bottles, cut off the tops, and ground the edges smooth.

Ron remembers the scarcity of those times: "Just before first grade I got pneumonia and damn near died. My father was so tight—the kind of person who put in forty-watt bulbs rather than seventy-fives. He bought a bargain casket for me."

Fortunately, Ron recovered, and the pair found plenty to do together while growing up in Berkeley, California. The two hiked in the hills, dug tunnels in the back yard, flew kites,

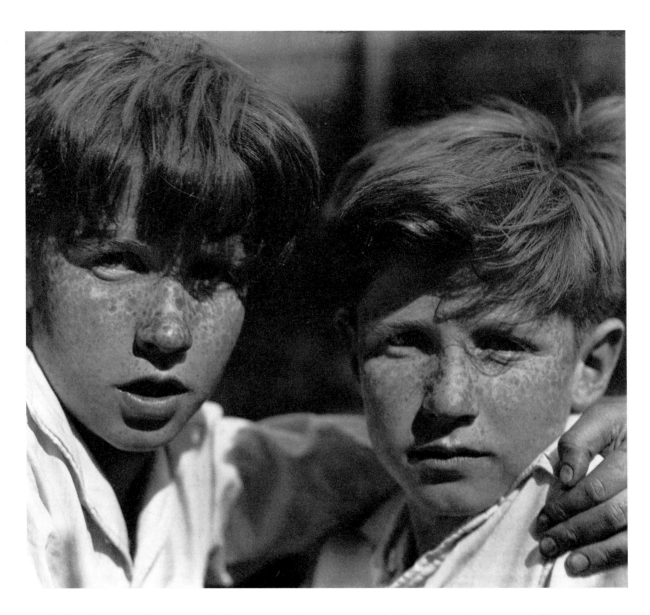

Pad (left) and Ron Partridge in 1927. Their mother, the famous photographer Imogen Cunningham, took this photograph.

climbed trees, and played baseball and an old-fashioned game called mumblety-peg, which is played by flipping a knife into the ground. They also ran around the neighborhood like little madmen and became known as the "devils."

Although they were identical twins and nearly impossible to tell apart, they developed different personalities and different way of dealing with their difficult dad. Their father wasn't just cheap. A harsh disciplinarian, he got very angry when the twins disobeyed him. Pad would try to go along with what his father wanted. Ron, on the other hand, was rebellious—he would tell his father off.

The twins kept these traits into their adult professional lives: Ron, the wild one, continuing to disregard authority, and taking a career that let him be his own boss; Pad the practical one, willing to work for others because it was in his interest to do so, taking a more conventional job. Ron couldn't wait to get out of high school, and didn't care much about his grades. Pad worked hard and prepared for university.

From age thirteen, Ron knew he would follow in the footsteps of his mother, Imogen Cunningham, who was a famous photographer. Early in his career he worked as an assistant to such important photographers as Ansel Adams and Dorothea Lange. He would also take his own pictures of cowboys at rodeos, which he sold to the same cowboys for seventy-five cents. Later he worked for photo agencies and periodicals but, being restless, never stayed in one place for too long. His bread and butter was photographing buildings for architects and magazines.

Ron married and had five children, but not much money. The family always worried that they'd lose their house. This didn't interfere with Ron's plans though. Two summers in a row he took his old Cadillac limousine, which he had spray painted metallic gold, put a double mattress across the back, and drove the whole family (and two dogs) from California to New York while he took pictures.

To this day, Ron uses his camera every day, experimenting with new ideas like printing photos on silk. Not photographing to him is like not breathing. But now he feels a special sense of urgency about his work because he's not sure how much longer he'll be able to do it.

Pad enjoyed photography too but didn't pursue it as a profession because, as he put it, "There's no money in it." He didn't want to live like his brother. He got his first paying work while still in high school, when the best jobs available to youngsters paid only twenty-five cents per hour. Pad lied about his age and got a man's job working two thousand feet down a coal mine as a "mucker" for sixty cents per hour. He would dig into piles of loose rock with a short-handled shovel, throw the rock over his shoulder into a ton cart, push the cart a quarter mile and then dump its contents. When that was accomplished he went through the whole process again—fifteen or twenty times. Wearing a carbide lamp on his head, he worked in a small, dark tunnel where he was exposed to underground gases and smoke from dynamite blasts. "It's not a job that a human should do," he says, "but I did it."

Once Pad was building a bridge across a thirty-foot open hole in a Nevada mine when the scaffolding broke and he plunged ninety-five terrifying feet. It seemed like certain death. Somehow, though every bone in his body was broken, he survived the fall—and perhaps even more amazing, he managed to crawl to an elevator shaft and ring the bell for help. He was taken to a nearby hospital, where a doctor with questionable qualifications put him in traction.

A week later, Ron, who was camping with his wife in Nevada for their honeymoon, showed up at the mine looking for his brother. The horrified miners thought they were seeing a ghost. "What are you doing here? You're practically dead!" they said.

Arriving at the hospital, Ron didn't like Pad's doctor—he had dirt underneath all his fingernails. Pad agreed, but the doctor wouldn't release him, so Ron and his wife waited till

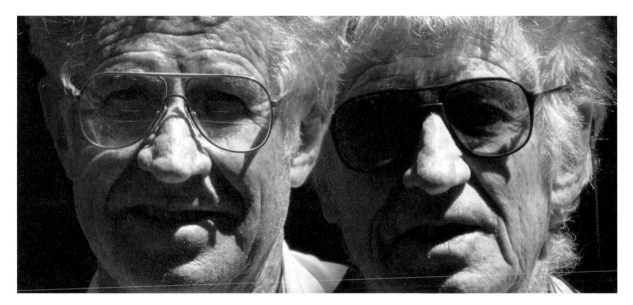

Pad (left) and Ron, in 1997—seventy years after their photo on page 22. Ron took this picture.

after dark and snuck Pad out of the hospital. Then they loaded him, on a stretcher, onto a train bound for Sacramento, where they put him in a better facility.

After attending college, Pad eventually worked his way up to much more pleasant and lucrative work as a mining engineer. He also became a clay specialist and traveled all over the world looking at mines to help companies determine the kinds of clay they could get from them. The clays were to be used for industry and even for cat litter.

Ron and Pad remain good friends who respect each other's differences. Ron still laughs at what he considers his brother's willingness to obey authority. "But," Ron says, "he's accomplished more in the world in that way than I have by doing the opposite."

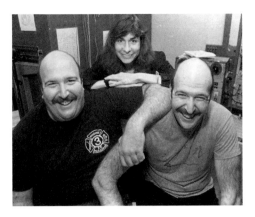

separated at birth

Imagine that someone shows up at your door one day. You don't know this person, but you could almost be looking at a mirror. You recognize those eyes, the hair, the nose, the mouth—they're yours! And when the person speaks, you say the same thing at the same time. The voice is yours too, and so is the body language. You feel a bit dizzy; you realize you've met your long lost twin, even though you never knew you had one.

This is the surreal experience of identical twins separated at birth and reunited much later in life.

• MY HEAD ON HIS SHOULDERS •

Here's the story of how twin volunteer firefighters were brought together after decades apart. In this surprising case it took fate and a third person—with a good eye—to reunite the pair.

In 1985 Jimmy Tedesco met Jerry Levey at a volunteer firefighters' convention in New

ABOVE: Twins Mark Newman (left) and Jerry Levey, who were separated at birth and reunited thirty-one years later, posing with twins researcher Nancy Segal, Ph.D.

Jersey. It was strange: Jerry looked like somebody—a lot like somebody—Jimmy knew. Jimmy learned that no, Jerry had no brother, that he was born on April 15, 1954, and that he was adopted.

Another volunteer firefighter friend of Jimmy's, Mark Newman, was the one who looked like Jerry. Mark, it turned out, was born the same day as Jerry. Same year too.

To have a little fun, Jimmy slyly arranged for the two to meet without revealing his plan. He traveled with Mark to Jerry's firehouse, approximately an hour's drive, telling him about some firefighting equipment there that they should see. Mark shook Jerry's hand and went off to find the equipment. Then Jimmy brought the two face-to-face again. This time a startled Mark exclaimed, "What's my bald head doing on his shoulders?"

Realizing they were twins who had been separated at birth, the shocked brothers compared everything about themselves. Although one was eighty pounds heavier, their heights (6'4"), sideburns, mustaches, bald heads, even the way the hair curled on their bodies, all matched perfectly. Looking back today on their reunion, Jerry says, "It was the twilight zone."

In addition to their firefighting careers, the thirty-two-year-old brothers had similar professions—Mark installed fire suppression systems and Jerry installed burglar alarm systems. They had the same favorite beer—Budweiser—and both held their beer mugs with their pinkies on the bottom. They both liked to eat their meat very rare. Finally, their scores on an intelligence test were only two points apart.

Stories of twins separated at birth may fascinate us, but they are also of great interest to scientists, who consider twins a "living laboratory." This is because they provide important clues in the age-old nature-vs.-nurture debate. They help answer the question, Are our personalities and our bodies formed more by the genes we inherit from our parents (nature) or by the environment in which we grew up and our experiences in it (nurture)? For instance, if you have an optimistic outlook, is it because you were born that way or because you grew up in a loving family and have always been treated well?

Identical twins share the same set of genes, while fraternal twins do not. By comparing the two types of twins, biologists and psychologists hope to determine whether various physical characteristics and personality traits are caused by genes, the environment, or a combination of both.

Here's how it works: if identical twins are more likely to share a trait than fraternal twins, that trait is thought to have a strong genetic component. Some examples of genetically influenced characteristics are: amount of body fat, religiousness, optimism and pessimism, alcoholism, and attention deficit disorder. Identical twins are more likely than others, for instance, to have the same amount of body fat.

When identical twins like Mark and Jerry are separated at birth and find each other later in life, they are especially valuable to scientists. Since they grew up in different environments, when they share traits, the cause is more than likely genetic.

• FRIENDS FOREVER •

In 1957 two girls were born to a seventeen-year-old unwed mother. The teen's father insisted that the girls, who were identical twins, be put up for adoption. The sisters ended up with different families, and grew up a few hours apart from each other in small towns in the Midwest. (It is not a standard practice now to split up twins for adoption, but it used to happen occasionally.)

Neither girl knew she had a twin; their adoptive families didn't know this either. Yet the girls, Stephanie Curry and Martha (Marti) Botsch, seemed to feel each other's absence from the time they were separated. They both cried a lot when moved to their adoptive homes, and the feeling of loss continued as they grew up apart. "It's an inner gnawing . . . and every day you wake up with it," Stephanie said. The two were reunited thirty-eight years later, after Marti undertook a search for her birth mother and discovered she had a twin; it turned out that for all those years Marti shared an "unsettling feeling" of missing something. But that's not all they shared.

"The first time I talked to Martha, it was like I'd known her my whole life," says Stephanie. When they met, in September 1995, at a restaurant located between their homes, each brought the other a gift. Eerily, it was the same gift, a little magnet with these words: "Sisters from the very start. Friends forever from the heart."

Staying at their birth mom's house soon after their reunion, they took off their clothing to compare themselves. "I had to see with my own two eyes that we were identical," says Marti.

They discovered that they had both had their tonsils out at seven years of age and both sparkled in spelling bees. A look at their high school photos shows their appearance to be exactly the same—even the way they wore their hair. Both had married in their early twenties and divorced in their mid-thirties.

The sisters were studied at the University of Minnesota's Center for Twin and Adoption Research, founded by Thomas J. Bouchard, Ph.D. Research there has revealed many amazing stories of twins separated at birth and reunited as adults. When scientists asked Marti and Stephanie individually to rank ten words or phrases in order of personal importance, each put "inner peace " at the top. And since they found each other, they both seem to have more of that quality. Stephanie sums it up this way: "I know who I am now. . . . And know that . . . there's nothing ever going to separate us again."

• the angel of death •

Sadly, the interest in twins and genetics was behind one of the darkest episodes in the history of twins. The tragedy occurred in Nazi Germany. The Nazis believed that by better understanding genetics, they could further their goal of creating an Aryan "super-race." Because identical twins are a genetic match, Nazi doctors believed them valuable in achieving this understanding. (Fraternal twins were also of interest, although less so.)

Between 1943 and 1945, Dr. Josef Mengele ran cruel experiments on 1,500 pairs of twins—mostly young children—at a concentration camp in Poland. Mengele was called the "Angel of Death" because he loved to choose people for execution in the gas chambers. Most of his twins were separated by force from their parents—who were later slaughtered or perished in the barbaric conditions of the camp—to be used as guinea pigs in Nazi research. This was the fate of twin Eva Mozes. She survived the ordeal along with her sister, Miriam, and many years later described her experience in the book *Children of the Flames*:

> We were always naked during the experiments.
> We were marked, painted, measured, observed. Boys and girls were together. It
> was all so demeaning. There was no place to hide, no place to go.
> They compared every part of our body with that of our twin. The tests would last
> for hours.

In the name of "science," Mengele also performed this grisly procedure on a number of sets of twins: He would subject one twin in a pair to X-rays, blood transfusions, and injections with disease-causing germs. Later the pair was executed so doctors could compare the organs in their bodies.

Many of the twins who survived met again forty years later in 1984 at an emotional reunion in Tel Aviv, Israel. They also traveled to Jerusalem for a three-day hearing on Mengele's war crimes and to Poland for a tour of their former concentration camp.

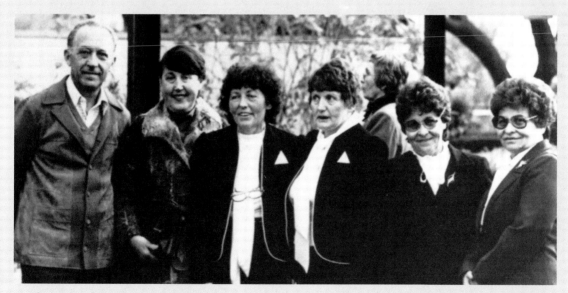

Three sets of twins who survived Nazi experiments met at a reunion in Tel Aviv, Israel: (left to right) Kalman Bar-On and his sister Yehadit Keren, Hedva Katz and Leah Feirstein, Eva Kor and Miriam Czaigher

• THE GIGGLE TWINS •

Another amazing twin story involves two British women, Barbara Herbert and Daphne Good-ship, who came to be known as the Giggle Twins. As infants these twins were adopted into different families when their mother committed suicide. They were reunited after forty years.

Though they had never met before, they had all this in common: they both grew up near London; quit school at fourteen; fell down stairs at fifteen, leaving each with weak ankles; and worked in local government. At sixteen they both met at a Town Hall dance the men they'd later marry. They had miscarriages in the same month, then gave birth to two boys and a girl. They both liked cold coffee, couldn't stand the sight of blood, and were scared of heights. Both had dyed their hair the same color in their youths. When they met, they were each wearing a jacket of brown velvet and a cream-colored dress. Each habitually pushed up her nose with her palm, and each had independently nicknamed this tick "squidging."

Interviewed separately by Thomas Bouchard, they told him the same lie: that they wanted to be opera singers. "Neither of us can sing a note," Barbara later confessed, and then both twins had a fit of giggling. It was the way they had of laughing continuously in each other's presence that earned them their nickname.

Why did these twins, who had different adoptive parents and grew up apart, have these bizarre things in common? Well, some of it may be coincidence, but several of the things the Giggle Twins have in common are related to traits known to have strong genetic components: taste in food, clothing, and choice of career. It's a little spooky,

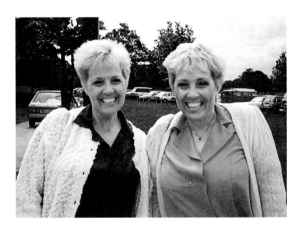

The Giggle Twins

32

if you think you have free will (make your own choices), to realize there is something inside you—part of your biological makeup—that greatly influences many things you do.

• BIZARRE SIMILARITIES •

Among the first twins to be studied at the University of Minnesota were Jim Lewis and Jim Springer. They were adopted at four weeks old by different parents, who lived seventy miles apart in Ohio, and reunited thirty-nine years later in 1979. Their bizarre similarities are the stuff of twin legend. Both twins were named Jim; married a woman named Linda; divorced her, and got remarried to a Betty; were raised with an adopted brother named Larry; in childhood, owned a dog called Toy; had worked part time as a deputy sheriff; were interested in mechanical drawing and carpentry; liked math most in school, spelling least; and vacationed at the same Florida Beach. Also, Springer named his first son James Allan while Lewis chose the name James Alan. "We even use the same slang," Lewis said after their reunion. "A lot of times, I'll start to say something and he'll finish it."

Because of the striking similarities discovered between identical twins reared apart, the nature-vs.-nurture debate has been tipping in nature's favor in recent years. But that doesn't mean genes control everything about us. Rather, experts believe that genes have a strong influence on our behaviors. Indeed, some identical twins are very different, and they illustrate the importance of the "nurture" side of the equation.

In one case, a pair of identical twin brothers raised together took vastly different paths in their lives. Today one of them, Conrad, is proficient in the martial arts, is dedicated to his own health, and works as a private detective. His brother, Perry, sadly, is a homeless alcoholic. It turns out that alcoholism, a genetically influenced disease, runs in the family. Conrad believes his brother turned to alcohol partly because he couldn't accept his wife's sudden death.

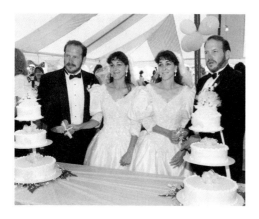

more amazing stories

• WE THEE WED •

It doesn't happen very often, but it does happen: two sets of twins fall in love and get married. Sometimes all four end up living together. That's how it went with twins Phil and Doug Malm, who married Jena and Jill Lassen (in that order).

The identical pairs met in 1991—the men were thirty-four, the women, twenty-four—at the annual Twins Day Festival in Twinsburg, Ohio. Twins gather there by the thousands to compete in "Most Alike" contests, to celebrate twinship, and to meet other twins. A few years later they got married at another Twins Day Festival—a double wedding with three thousand guests! Looking back at the ceremony, says Phil, the brothers remembered saying, "Will you marry me?" But a videotape tells a different story. They really said, "Will you marry us?" All four moved into the same house in Moscow, Idaho, where Doug and Phil run a carpentry business and their wives work as day-care teachers.

ABOVE: Phil and Jena Malm (left) and Jill and Doug Malm cutting cakes at their wedding during the Twins Day Festival in Twinsburg, Ohio, August 1993

Sometimes twins pair off with other twins because they find it difficult to date singletons. Often a nontwin will not understand the twin bond and will feel jealous. Or, as in Jena's case, a twin may feel jealous when her sister-twin is dating and she is not. For these reasons, Doug, Phil, Jill and Jena were each resigned to remaining single before they met their future spouses. But why did each twosome make their household a foursome? These twins were so close, Jill said, that "there would be no point living apart, since we'd always just end up in each other's houses anyway."

Jill and Jena are the closer of the twin pairs. That might be because they were treated as one person when they were children. The two share a car and go everywhere together—shopping, attending craft shows, visiting friends—while each of their husbands has his own van and goes off on his own. Jill and Jena also have identical mannerisms, facial expressions, and posture, and will cross their legs as well as speak at the same time.

Another set of twins who met their match at Twins Day are Cal and Ali McGregor. Cal married Jim Stanch, Ali, his twin, Jeff Stanch. As with the Malm couples, firstborn married firstborn, secondborn married secondborn, and all four moved in together.

Cal and Ali had each been previously

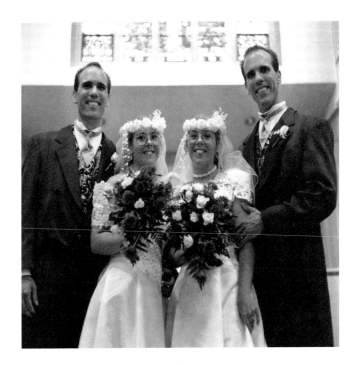

Jim, Cal, Ali, and Jeff (left to right) on their wedding day engaged to singletons, but neither relationship worked out. Says Ali, "Cal's fiancé was very intimidated by our [twin] bond.... My fiancé wanted me to himself all the time and would try to split me and Cal up."

Most people in married twin sets don't consider their spouses interchangeable. They have very different feelings toward their spouse and their spouse's twin, and could never switch partners. They say their in-law is like a sibling or friend, not like a husband or wife. "I don't find Ali attractive in the same way as Cal," explains Jim. "She looks different to me."

Cal says that if they decided to have kids, "It would be nice to have them around the same time." And married identical twin pairs can do something impossible for anyone else. The children of one pair will share, on average, half of their genes with the other pair's children. They will not only be cousins; they will be genetic siblings as well!

• INCREDIBLE TWIN TEAMS •

Twins, who often know each other better than the closest husbands and wives, can make powerful teams. Two pairs—the Hollenbeck brothers and the Mendez brothers—have accomplished great things through their cooperation.

One morning when he was fourteen, Scot Hollenbeck got on his brand-new Schwinn bike and took off down a two-lane country road for swim practice. His twin brother, Sean, who usually went with Scot, decided to stay in bed. Soon after beginning his trip, Scot shifted gears and then, suddenly, a car hit him, leaving him lying in a drizzle. When he woke up, his first concern was about the condition of his bike. But his body was severely twisted, and when his mother came to him, he could tell from her face that something was extremely wrong.

Scot was taken to the hospital, and his parents thought he was going to die. Sean, left home alone, went to the accident site and picked up pieces of the destroyed bike. Now twenty-eight, he says, "I can remember being really angry at myself for not being there for my brother, and punching the garage wall until my fist was all bloody."

Scot survived after seven hours of surgery. His spinal cord was severed and he was paralyzed below the waist; he would never walk again. He began a difficult rehabilitation. The idea that he could no longer pursue the sports he loved so much depressed him. Watching Sean from the sidelines, he says, "One part of me was so excited for my brother when he made a tackle in football, but the other half looked at the wheelchair and got angry."

Sean was depressed too. He went from doing everything with his brother to doing nothing. He felt guilty that he couldn't help more.

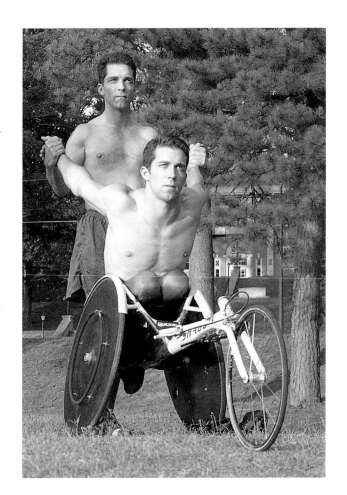

Sean and Scot (front) Hollenbeck

But Scot kept a positive attitude, and eventually he realized he could get back into sports—that while he could no longer run, he still could race. The first inspiration came four days after the accident. Watching TV from his hospital bed, he saw an eight-hundred-meter wheelchair race at a 1984 Olympic event.

With the aid of his brother, Scot eventually became an Olympic wheelchair racer himself, winning a silver medal. And Sean became a doctor, so he would never be helpless again in the face of his brother's problems. He spends much of his time teaching people about disabilities. He says of Scot, "We're part of each other, and to see him accomplish his goals and be the best in the world just makes me glow."

In another accomplished twin team, both siblings are doctors. Twin Los Angeles surgeons Robert and Ralph Mendez can work together as few others can. When they perform an operation, says Ralph, "It's sort of automatic. We can go through a whole surgery and not say a word. It's just like four hands out of the same brain. We can operate in about half the time of somebody else." The Mendez brothers, who work at the leading edge of kidney transplantation, said their twinship also serves them when they work different shifts. They look so much alike that their patients are comforted by the illusion their doctor is always on the floor. These days it's unusual for the two to perform surgery together—they now have seven other partners on their team. But when a transplant is from one living relative to another, Ralph will remove a healthy kidney from the donor and Robert will transfer it into the recipient.

• READING MINDS •

When a twin dies in a horrible accident, does the surviving twin suffer more because of their mysterious connection?

Some people believe that identical twins can communicate with each other from far away without talking. Martha Burke thought she and her twin sister had this kind of ESP (extrasensory perception). Burke tried to sue an airline for the pain she suffered during a 1977 plane crash—even though she was thousands of miles from the accident. It was her twin sister who died when her plane collided with another on a runway in the Canary Islands.

Burke claimed that at the moment the tragedy occurred, she felt an intense burning sensation in her breast and abdomen. She felt as though her body had been cut in half. Now she believed that the accident had caused long-term damage to her. However, the judge in the case decided that U.S. law does not recognize this kind of injury.

There have been other similar reports of ESP between twins. In one case, a man in Heapham, England, named Percy Black said, "I feel something is wrong in Sheffield." He died moments later. As it turned out, his twin brother, Cecil, had collapsed and died at his club in Sheffield earlier the same day.

Then there's the story told by a judge about his school days with his twin brother. On one test the twins' answers were so similar that the teachers decided to separate them next time. But on their next exams, in Latin, the twins wrote with the same words and the same grammar. To top it off, they made the same errors. At the start of the test, one twin had felt unable to begin writing and could not explain why. It turned out that his brother in the other room had been delayed by some paperwork. Once this was taken care of, both young men began to write at the same time.

Of course, many scientists don't believe in ESP—whether in twins or anyone else. They would say that these stories could be explained by coincidence rather than by anything "mysterious."

• THE SECRET LANGUAGE •

When they were children, the identical twins Gracie and Ginny Kennedy made up names for each other: Poto and Cabengo. They would speak to each other like this:

"Cabengo, padem manibadu peetu."

"Pinit, Poto."

They understood one another perfectly. They would use their language to do things like name the objects around them in the house. Of course no one else knew what they were saying—to others it sounded as though they were from another planet. So when talking with adults, they spoke English or German (their grandmother's language) and made signs with their bodies. When adults tried to learn the twins' special language, Poto and Cabengo resisted.

Language experts listened to the twins' conversations. They found that it contained made-up words as well as English and German words. They have discovered that many young identical twins have a private language. They're not sure why this happens, but it may have something to do with the twin relationship and the similarities in twins' language development. Also, most twins who develop their own language had little contact with other kids early in life.

• THE DARK SIDE •

Not all twin relationships are models of cooperation and support. Like any human relationship, a twin relationship can be unhealthy. This was spectacularly the case with June and Jennifer Gibbons, who grew up in West Wales, Great Britain.

As children, these identical twins spoke only to each other in what seemed to be a private language. They wouldn't converse with others, earning them the nickname the "Silent Twins." Incredibly, at eleven years of age, they had never talked at school or to their father or siblings.

And their bizarre behavior didn't stop there—the twins could sometimes be seen marching with a kind of goose step, with one following ten yards behind the other, from the school playground all the way home.

At age thirteen they were moved to a special school. When authorities there decided to separate them from each other, the intensity of their love-hate relationship was put on display: They began fighting each other fiercely, ripping out each other's hair. According to June, her sister screamed, "She's mine! She's mine!"

June's psychiatrist, Tegwyn Williams, believed the twins' problems came from their not being accepted by the people where they lived. Their parents were from Barbados, in the Caribbean, and the twins were black and had West Indian accents. They also had bad speech impediments. It's possible their troubles were caused partly by a negative reaction of the overwhelmingly white community where they lived in Wales. This may have caused them to withdraw further into their private twin world.

The twins' antisocial behavior escalated as they grew older, until at age nineteen they burned down a tractor store. When police caught them soon after that attempting to torch a college building, the pair were confined to Broadmoor, a maximum-security mental hospital. In her diary there, June wrote of Jennifer, "This sister of mine, a dark shadow robbing me of sunlight, is my one and only torment."

The two were released after more than ten years at Broadmoor. Jennifer died less than twelve hours later. She had suffered from a "roaring inflammation with the heart muscle completely destroyed," according to the pathologist.

Later, June said she'd been "trapped in twinship" and "born in captivity," and described their relationship as one in which she was the more independent sibling, who wanted to be free of her more needy sister. There were many theories as to what could have caused Jennifer's death, but June has definite ideas on the subject. She claimed that Jennifer died so June could be free. "She released me," said June.

A sick relationship is one thing, but some people have committed terrible crimes against their twin. Twins have even tried to murder twins. At age twenty-two, Jeen Young Han

(Gina), labeled the "evil twin" in news reports, tried to have her sister, Sunny (the "good twin"), killed. These Korean twins had seemed to get along with each other as teens, and both were valedictorians at their San Diego County high school. After their graduation, though, they started fighting. Gina stole a car and credit cards from Sunny, who had her sister imprisoned. Later Gina paid two teenagers to kill Sunny; she planned to take on her identity. The attempt failed, and Gina was arrested.

Fortunately, stories this extreme, while powerful, are rare. Most people find it difficult even to contemplate their twin's death, let alone bringing it about by their own hand.

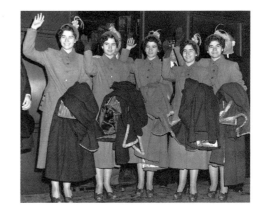

multiples

Being parents of twins is a challenge, but what about multiplying the brood—say, by a factor of two? This tremendous responsibility faced Jim Wills and Kelly Curry-Wills of Plant City, Florida, mom and dad to quadruplets. To say that their lives were changed would be an understatement.

Even though they get help from members of their church, friends, and relatives, they still face countless diaper changes and four hungry mouths. So, not surprisingly, they're home a lot. As Kelly put it when the quads were one and she and her husband were thirty-nine, "Every now and then Jim and I go out. One of the first times, we just rode around with some friends. But a trip to Wal-Mart is like going to Europe." And, like any new parents, only more so, they're tired a lot: Kelly falls asleep anytime she tries to read.

But it's all worth it. Especially since the babies—big Royce, brave Bruce, little Zoe, and their leader Hal—have happy temperaments and smile a lot. "I would not trade a minute of this," Kelly said.

ABOVE: **The sixteen-year-old Dionne quintuplets leave New York City, 1950**

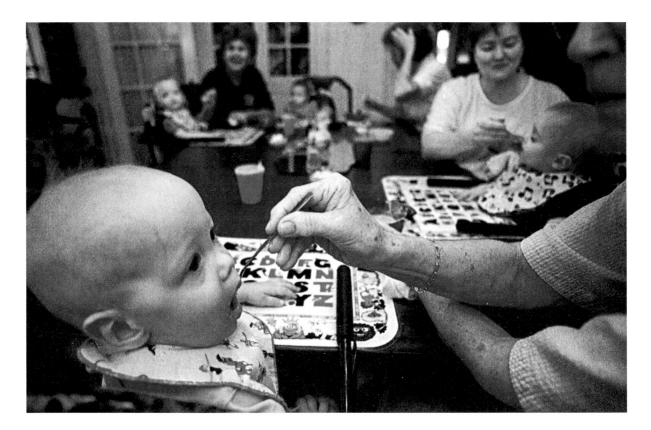

The Curry-Wills quadruplets, Royce, Bruce, Zoe, and Hal, age one

The number of multiple births—triplets, quadruplets, or more—has increased about six-fold in the last twenty years. This is for the same reason that twin births have increased: women putting off childbirth until their late thirties and then, in many cases, using fertility treatments.

A woman may resort to a fertility treatment after years of trying—and failing—to get pregnant. One option is to take fertility drugs, which stimulate the release of eggs into the uterus. If more than one egg is released and the eggs are fertilized, the woman may have twins or more. The drugs end in twins for 20 percent of users, and in triplets or more for an additional 5 percent.

A woman may also opt to use in-vitro fertilization (IVF), as Kelly Curry-Wills did. In this procedure, eggs are removed from a woman's body, fertilized with sperm in a dish, and then implanted in the woman's uterus. Because not all of the fertilized eggs are expected to "take," doctors often implant several. The patient risks the possibility that many of the eggs will be successful, and she will become pregnant with multiples. After years of not being able to conceive, this is what happened to Kelly Curry-Wills and what occurs with many other women as well.

Fertility treatments—which can be like a roll of the dice—have led to some extreme situations.

• SEVENTH HEAVEN •

When Bobbi McCaughey (pronounced "McCoy"), a seamstress who lived in Carlisle, Iowa, became pregnant after taking fertility drugs, her doctors could not believe their eyes. Six weeks into the pregnancy, an ultrasound machine revealed that she was, well, extremely pregnant. She was carrying seven fetuses.

The odds against delivering seven healthy babies—septuplets—are high. In 1985 Patricia Frustaci of Orange, California, had seven babies. Sadly, one was stillborn, three died within nineteen days, and the three survivors suffered from cerebral palsy and retardation.

Because of such hazards, doctors gave Bobbi and her husband, Kenny, a choice. If they didn't want to go through such a risky pregnancy, they could choose a procedure called "selective termination." This would mean that several of the fetuses would be eliminated to save the remaining ones.

The McCaughey's decision wasn't difficult for them: the proposed procedure was a form of abortion, and their religious beliefs prohibited this act. They would trust God to see them through.

Doctors soon ordered Bobbi to bed for the duration of the pregnancy. Most multiple pregnancies end in premature births, which exposes the babies to more health risks. Bobbi's physicians hoped that if she stayed in bed and took medication to delay labor contractions, she would carry her babies for a period long enough to ensure their health. She lasted almost thirty weeks, longer than expected.

On November 19, 1997, Bobbi McCaughey underwent a cesarean section and made history as a team of forty doctors pulled seven babies, heavier (2.5 to 3.4 pounds) and healthier than had been dreamed of, from her body. First Hercules (so nicknamed because he had supported the weight of the others inside the uterus), also known as Kenneth, was brought into the world, followed by siblings Alexis May, Natalie Sue, Kelsey Ann, Brandon James, Nathan Roy, and Joel Steven. When doctors finally allowed the proud parents to hold Kenneth, Bobbi said, "It was incredible, I can't wait to hold all of them."

There was an outpouring of support in Carlisle. The McCaugheys had been living in a small house, and now needed much more room. So the mayor promised the family a plot of land, and businesses in the area offered to construct a new house for them, complete with appliances. A car company made them the gift of a large van, and their neighbors pitched in to help with the nuts and bolts of daily life with seven new babies and their toddler sister: laundry, cleaning, feeding, driving, baby sitting, etc. And several large corporations made big gifts: free diapers for life, baby food, even college scholarships.

• MULTIPLE HAZARDS •

It all sounds so wonderful—a miraculous birth, proud parents, community support. But for some people, there was something very wrong with this picture. Some doctors and other ex-

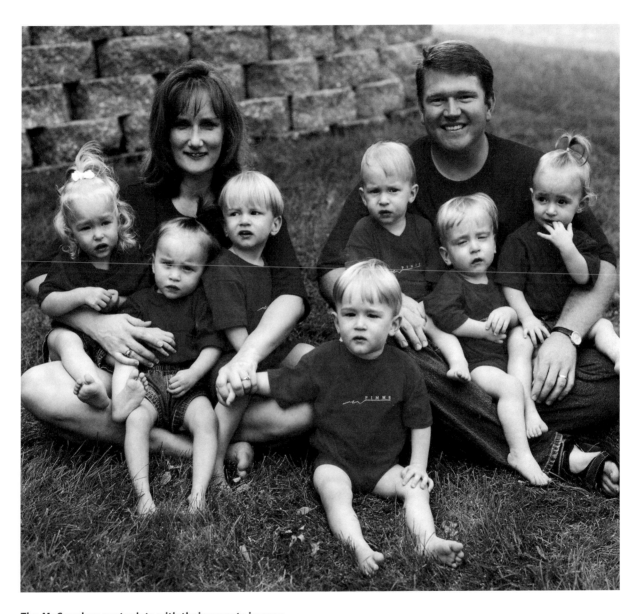

The McCaughey septuplets with their parents in 1999

perts worry that the McCaughey's story makes it look too easy and encourages the trend toward more multiples.

They point to the difficulties and dangers that haunt multiple births. For one thing, carrying them in the womb is extremely difficult and uncomfortable for the mother. A woman's uterus is designed for a load of six to eight pounds. When someone carries more, as happens with multiples, she may have trouble walking or breathing, and her heart may be stressed.

Toward the end of a pregnancy, mothers are given drugs to delay labor contractions so the babies won't be too premature. The drugs can temporarily cause nausea, irritability, slurred speech, and even partial blindness. Also, mothers of multiples face a higher risk of death during pregnancy or delivery from strokes or bleeding.

Multiples have health risks, and the higher the number, the greater the risk. This made philosopher Jennifer McCrickerd wonder whether people would have still viewed Bobbi and Kenny McCaughey positively if their babies had been stillborn. If they survive, multiples are more likely to suffer from cerebral palsy, brain damage, blindness, bowel and kidney problems, mental retardation, and other developmental problems. Birthing and caring for them is expensive—the McCaughey pregnancy is estimated to have had a million-dollar price tag—and most multiples don't inspire the community and corporate support that record-breaking births receive.

If the cost and health problems don't sink parents, the housekeeping, diapering, and other chores might. One father of quintuplets, overwhelmed by the responsibility, killed himself. A doctor summed it up this way: "It is an injustice to children to be born in litters." And for some, the costs involved also make it an injustice to the whole society—which channels enormous resources so one family can have children.

The McCaugheys were the first couple ever to have surviving septuplets. About one year later another couple became parents of octuplets—*eight* children. The mother, twenty-seven-year-old Nkem Chukwu, a woman from Nigeria who was living in Houston, carried her babies for about the same amount of time as Bobbi McCaughey. But they weighed much less—eleven ounces to two pounds—and doctors feared for their lives.

Nkem, who also turned down selective reduction, endured a difficult period at the end of her pregnancy. She was confined to bed for six weeks—and for the final two and a half weeks, when doctors tilted the head of her bed toward the floor to take pressure off her lower body, she lay virtually upside down. Also, to give the babies more room to grow, she gave up eating for a while and was fed intravenously.

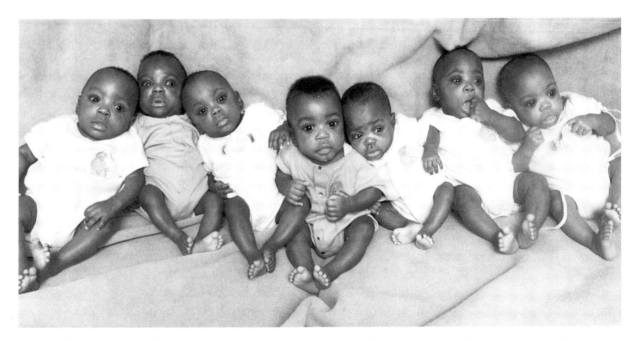

The surviving seven of the Chukwu octuplets, age 7 months. Left to right: Chima, Ikem, Ebuka, Jioke, Gorom, Echerem, and Chidi

As in the McCaughey multiple birth, individuals and companies donated money and various products—including cribs and baby wipes. The father, Iyke Louis Udobi, made a public announcement expressing appreciation for this support and saying, "Our family is very excited and grateful to God."

Sadly, illustrating the health hazards of this kind of birth, the smallest baby—named Odera—died within a week. And illustrating the financial hazards, the hospital charges for the surviving babies were $250,000 each.

The McCaugheys have had some problems of their own. About two years after their septuplets were born, they revealed that Nathan and Alexis suffered from birth defects causing muscular weakness and tightness. This made it difficult for them to crawl or walk. The parents said they were hopeful that the problems could eventually be overcome with physical therapy and other medical treatment.

• AN IMPOSSIBLE CHOICE •

Sometimes doctors know in advance that some of the fetuses in a multiple birth will die if the mother carries them all. Because of this and other hazards of multiple births, more and more women are faced with these difficult and unexpected ethical questions: Should they deliberately have one or more of their fetuses aborted by a doctor? What if the only way to save some fetuses is to kill the rest?

The "selective termination" procedure is most often done between nine and twelve weeks into the pregnancy. A fetus—about an inch long at this point—is chosen to be removed, based on how easy it will be for the doctor to reach. The doctor then passes a needle through the mother's abdomen and injects a chemical into this fetus that kills it. Usually patients will choose to eliminate all but two fetuses. In addition to the ethical problems some people have with this procedure, there is also a practical one: women who go through with it face a much greater chance that their entire pregnancy will be lost than do women who refuse it.

One woman who opted for selective termination was given the false name Charlotte by a newspaper to protect her privacy. She was small (112 lbs.), but was pregnant with six fetuses. Before becoming pregnant, she had received fertility treatments for nine years. Finally, in-vitro fertilization worked, but too well. A doctor told Charlotte that her babies definitely wouldn't all survive, informed her about selective reduction, and suggested that she reduce to twins.

Charlotte and her husband contemplated their situation for a long weekend. Her religious beliefs went against selective reduction, but there didn't seem to be any way around it. In the end she opted to carry the highest possible number: four fetuses. She wept after having two of the fetuses eliminated.

After thirty weeks—two months shy of the time a mother usually carries a single baby—she gave birth to quadruplets, almost suffering a stroke at the end. The babies grew into four healthy toddlers, but at times she still thinks about how the other two would have turned out.

• THE BIG SHOW •

The risks to their health and the enormous financial burden of raising multiples are not the only problems. Famous multiples like the McCaugheys may also lose their privacy. They face the possibility that their lives "could turn into a big show," as Kenny McCaughey put it.

This is just what happened to the Dionne quintuplets, who were born in Ontario, Canada, in 1934. The five children—Annette, Yvonne, Cécile, Marie, and Emilie—were unusual not

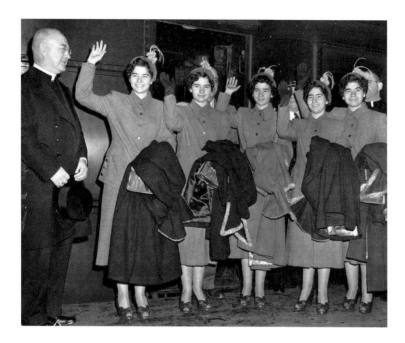

The sixteen-year-old Dionne quintuplets leave New York City, 1950: (left to right) Annette, Cécile, Yvonne, Marie, and Emilie

just for being quintuplets, but because they were identical quints who all developed from a single fertilized egg. It was the first time this had ever happened, and it hasn't happened since.

When Elzire Dionne gave birth to these girls, she and her husband, Oliva, were in a desperate situation. They already were raising five other children, and since they were poor farmers living in the middle of the Great Depression, it seemed impossible for them to feed so many mouths. To raise money, they agreed to allow the baby girls to be exhibited at the Chicago World's Fair in exchange for a percentage of what people paid to see them. But when the public heard about this scheme to use the quints as a tourist attraction, there was an outcry and the Ontario government stepped in, taking custody of the girls to protect them from exploitation.

They were soon moved into a nursery the government built across the road from the Dionnes' home. Later, sensing an opportunity to bring much needed money into the area as well as distract people from gloomy economic times, government authorities hatched their own plan to put the quints on display. The nursery was expanded into a kind of human zoo called Quintland. The Dionnes would spend their days playing in a horseshoe-shaped observatory that let paying crowds watch them through screened glass.

They were a sensation: For nine years, thousands of people came to Quintland every day to gawk at the Dionnes, whose pictures also appeared on products ranging from soft drinks to typewriters. Meanwhile, the quints' parents were allowed to see them for a half hour a day at most.

When they were finally returned to their family, they were like strangers. Tensions grew between the quints and their other siblings. The father was accused of sexually abusing the five girls, and they moved out at age eighteen.

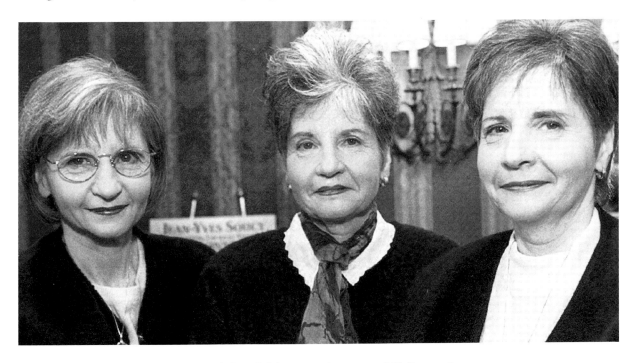

The three surviving Dionne quintuplets: (left to right) Yvonne, Annette, and Cécile, age 63

Because, they say, of mismanagement, the quints saw little of the money made off of them. Two of them suffered from health problems and died at an early age. As the others grew older, they suffered illness and poverty. Eventually they sued the Canadian government for exploiting them. In March 1998 the government settled with the Dionnes, awarding the sisters $2.8 million for their suffering.

When the McCaughey septuplets were born, the Dionne sisters, feeling "a natural affinity and tenderness" for them, sent their parents a letter. In it they said that their own "lives were forever altered by our childhood experience." They also wrote, "We hope your children receive more respect than we did. Their fate should be no different from that of other children. Multiple births should not be confused with entertainment, nor should they be an opportunity to sell products."

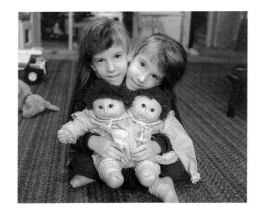

conjoined twins

Abigail and Brittany Hensel are ten-year-old identical twin sisters. Like other twins, they have their similarities—they both like to play piano and to sing "I'm a Little Teapot"—and their differences—Abby's wardrobe is daring, Britty's is demure. But there is something quite unusual about them, something that separates them from almost all other identical twins, and that is the fact that they are not separated. Rather, they are *conjoined*, which means they are physically attached. Specifically, they share one torso, two arms and two legs. Everywhere Abby goes—she's the one on the right—Britty goes with her, and vice versa.

• UNITED FROM BIRTH •

Twins who are conjoined, like the Hensels, come from the same single fertilized egg (zygote), have the same genes, and are the same sex. Identical twins are created when a zygote splits soon after fertilization. Conjoined twins occur when this split is delayed until after the

ABOVE: Abigail and Brittany Hensel in 1996—holding their conjoined-twin doll

thirteenth day. They are identical twins who were not completely separated in the womb, and who remain attached after birth.

Conjoined twins have always fascinated people. They may have been the inspiration for such mythological beings as the Roman god Janus, who had two faces, and the Greek centaurs, who were half man and half horse.

Today their presence challenges us as we strive to accept those who have disabilities or unusual appearances. Though they have at times been treated as monsters, conjoined twins want the same things from life that the rest of us do, and often they are able to get it.

First, some basic facts. Conjoined twins are three times more likely to be female than male and are most common in Africa and India. They are rare. Fewer than a dozen pairs live in the United States today. In the womb they often don't survive, possibly because the mother's body rejects them and they are lost in a miscarriage. Three-quarters of them are either stillborn or die soon after birth. They account for only one in 200,000 live births.

Such births often take parents by surprise, because there may be no clues during a pregnancy that a woman is carrying conjoined twins. Many forms of conjoining are possible. Some twins are closely united, and may even share bodily organs, such as a liver. Others may be attached by a small piece of flesh. But all of them are joined in one way or another and, unless they can be separated, will spend every moment of their days together.

Scientists classify conjoined twins according to where they are attached. The most common type is *thoracopagus* twins, which make up about 35 percent of all conjoined twins. They are joined at the chest. *Omphalopagus*, the next most common (30 percent), are connected from the waist to the lower breastbone. *Pygopagus* twins (19 percent of conjoined twins) are united at their backsides, and their positioning is almost back-to-back.

A more unusual type is the "parasitic twin," a small twin who is attached to and depends on the more normal sibling. The dependent twin may, for instance, be a head and arms joined to the abdomen of the normal twin.

Why does conjoining happen? Modern-day researchers say a variety of things may lead to delayed egg division, which causes conjoining. These include genetics, the environment, and exposure to toxic substances. But instances of conjoining were recorded a thousand years ago, and historical explanations are far more colorful.

In 1495, for instance, people explained the birth in Europe of two baby girls joined at the forehead this way: when pregnant, their mother accidentally hit her head against another woman's head. Her fear reaction affected her fetus, causing the formation of conjoined twins.

Ambroise Paré, a surgeon who lived in the sixteenth century, said conjoined twins were "contrary to the common decree and order of nature." He believed they were the result of such forces as God's anger, the Devil, a woman having too small a uterus, wearing tight clothing, or sitting in a certain way during pregnancy. In the eighteenth century researchers theorized that conjoined twins were created when two separate twin embryos came together in the womb, or when one egg was fertilized by two sperm. A minority of scientists still think these may be valid theories.

• THE HISTORICAL RECORD •

Possibly the earliest recorded case of conjoining involved Mary and Eliza Chulkhurst of Biddenden, England, born in 1100 A.D. Joined at their lower backs, these sisters lived to be thirty-four years old. When one died, physicians, wanting to save her twin's life, offered to perform an operation to separate the two. However, the surviving twin was not interested and told the doctors, "As we came together, we will also go together." Her own death came hours later.

The Chulkhurst twins left twenty acres of land to a church in their parish, on the condi-

57

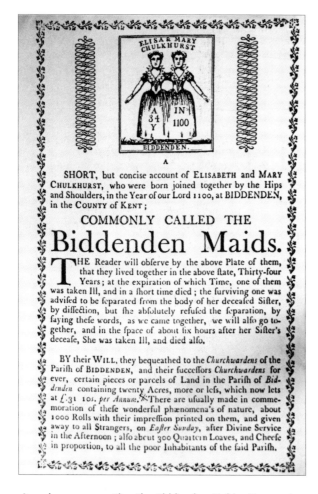

A card commemorating the Biddenden Maids, Mary and Eliza Chulkhurst, born 1100 A.D.

tion that income generated by rents go to feed the poor on Easter Sunday. To honor them for this gift, one thousand small dinner rolls stamped with their impression were distributed to the poor in Biddenden by the church on the same day (in addition to bread and cheese). This ritual lives on today, almost a millennium later.

The term "Siamese twin" comes from Chang and Eng Bunker, conjoined twins born in Siam (now Thailand) in 1811 to a half Chinese mother and a Chinese father. United at the lower chest by a tubular band of tissue (3¼ inches long and 1½ inches in diameter) connecting their livers, Chang and Eng eventually gained fame and fortune showing their unusual bodies at circuses and other performance stages.

At eighteen the two began a career as an attraction that took them to the United States, Canada, Cuba, and Europe. Their performances included acrobatic acts and displays of strength, and they'd also reveal their bodily connection to onlookers. In England they put on shows at the best-known places and even met members of the British royalty.

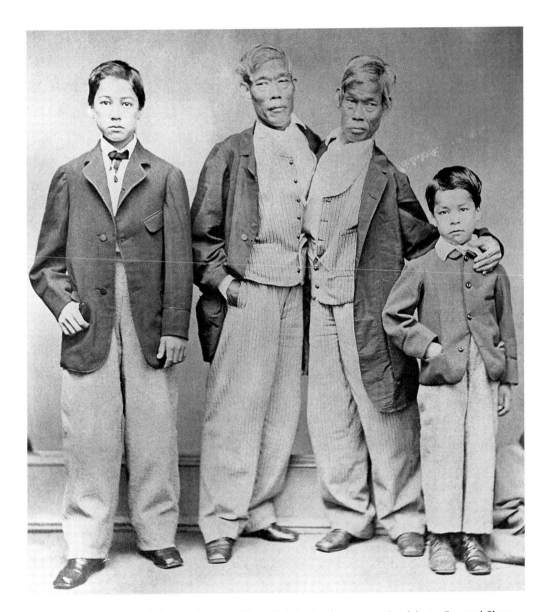

Chang and Eng Bunker with two of their children: (left to right) Eng's son Patrick, 15; Eng and Chang,
54; Chang's son Albert, 8

At twenty-eight, the brothers gave up touring for a while and became farmers in North Carolina. Four years later they each got married to the daughter of a clergyman—Eng to Sarah Ann Yates and Chang to her sister Adelaide. They kept two households and would alternate three-day visits to their own wives. Each got his turn as the decision-making twin in his own home. Over time the marriages would produce twenty-one children.

Curious doctors studied Chang and Eng to better understand their anatomy and the nature of their connection. At times the brothers considered surgery that would separate them, but they decided that the risks were too great, and that in any case, they had adapted well to their existing situation. In addition to their exhibition feats and their farming, they were skilled at shooting guns and could also run and swim.

One night in 1874 Eng awoke to find that his brother was dead. Eng died hours later. An autopsy revealed that Chang had died of a blood clot in his brain. The reason for Eng's death was unknown, but some doctors believed he might have died of fright. Doctors today believe his connection to his brother's corpse made him bleed to death.

Opinion is divided about Chang and Eng's influence on how the world views conjoined twins. In her book *Entwined Lives*, Nancy Segal wrote that it was unfortunate that the brothers' appearance as a circus attraction "lent freakish overtones to conjoined twins." But Laura Beardsley, who wrote the notes to the Mutter Museum (Philadelphia) exhibition on these twins, disagreed. She said Chang and Eng "changed the way society viewed conjoined twins and people with physical differences" by showing that their lives can be normal, with occupations, spouses, and children.

Several other conjoined twin pairs gained fame by becoming public attractions. Whether they did this of their own free will or not, there has always been an audience ready to pay to gawk at people considered freaks. In the mid-1800s, the North Carolina pygopagus (attached back-to-

60

back) girls Millie-Christine were put on display for money near age two. These conjoined twins were vulnerable not only because of their physical anomaly but because they were slaves. They were separated from their family early on by people seeking to profit from them. After being returned to their family, they were kidnapped by an exhibitor in New Orleans and eventually taken to London (where they charmed Queen Victoria); then once again they were returned to America and reunited with family.

Billed as the "Eighth Wonder of the World," Millie-Christine succeeded on stage back in the United States, where they performed even after the Civil War ended and they were freed from slavery. Appearing as the "Two-Headed Nightingale," they per-

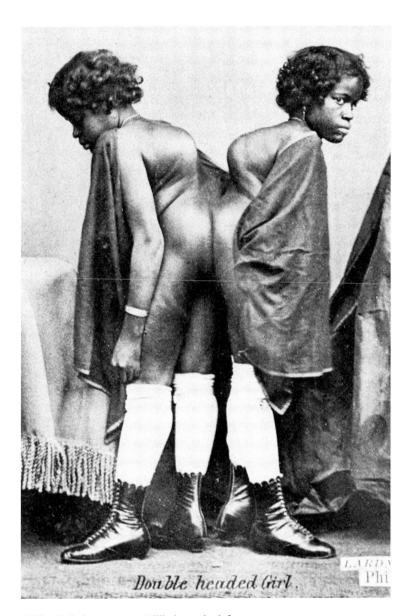

Double headed Girl.

Millie-Christine, age 20. Millie is on the left.

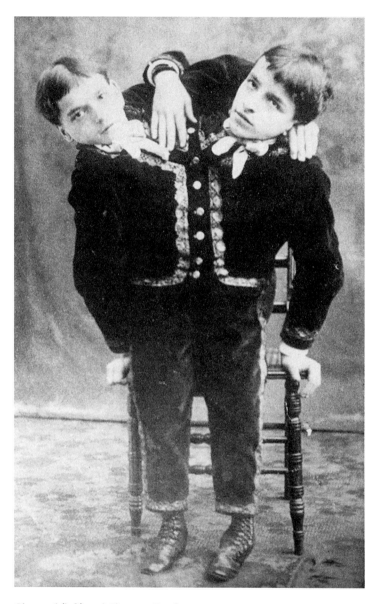

Giovanni (left) and Giacomo Tocci

formed a routine that included singing songs written for them and dancing as well.

The Tocci brothers, Giacomo and Giovanni, lived in Italy in the late 1800s and toured Europe and the United States as the "Blended Twins" or the "Two-Headed Boy." As the photo shows, their connection was extreme; while divided above the waist, they shared one abdomen and pelvis. Each brother controlled only one of their two legs, and they never mastered the coordination needed to walk without help. Each could write, though, and both were artistic. Like Chang and Eng, the Tocci brothers married sisters. After retiring from touring, they lived in seclusion near Venice.

Like Millie-Christine, Violet and Daisy Hilton of England were pygopagus twins. They were born in 1908 to an unmarried mother and raised by a tyrannical guardian, Mary Hilton. Mary held the twins against their wishes and made them perform on stage, singing, dancing, and playing musical instruments.

The twins eventually made a dramatic escape and took over their own careers. They performed in two movies—the 1932 classic *Freaks*, a tale of life in the circus, and *Chained for Life*, which posed a difficult but perhaps silly question: If one conjoined twin commits a murder, is it fair to send both siblings to jail?

Violet's desire to marry proved to be a problem. She and her fiancé were refused a marriage license several times because their union was considered immoral and indecent. The idea that Daisy would be an ever-present witness to Violet's lovemaking shocked authorities. Finally, they were permitted to wed in Texas. Although both sisters had husbands, the marriages did not last for long.

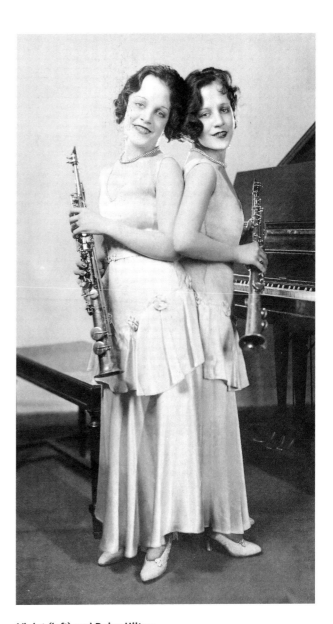

Violet (left) and Daisy Hilton

When their show-business careers ended in the 1960s, the twins moved to Charlotte, North Carolina, and worked as cashiers in a grocery store. They died from flu complications at sixty-one.

• THE DILEMMA OF SEPARATION •

About two hundred operations have been performed to separate conjoined twins, the earliest in the tenth century. The first successful attempt was made by a German doctor in 1689. He separated twins who were attached at the waist.

When conjoined twins are born ill, a difficult ethical problem may arise. It sometimes happens that only one twin has a chance of survival, and that chance depends on sacrificing the other. Parents may want to separate the twins surgically and try to save the stronger of them. This is what happened in the case of Amy and Angela Lakeberg, born in 1993.

The sisters were born joined from chest to belly; they shared a liver and a deformed heart. Their mother, Reitha Lakeberg, had known she was carrying conjoined twins with a low chance of surviving and had considered an abortion, but in the end, she said, "I couldn't get rid of my babies." The infants' health was so poor after birth, doctors wanted to take them off the ventilator that kept them alive.

But the Lakebergs instead found a hospital in Philadelphia where surgeons would separate the twins with the hope that their defective heart could be sufficiently repaired to allow one of them to live. Angela had the better chance, but even her odds of survival were less than one percent.

On the day of the surgery, nurses painted Angela's fingernails pink while they left Amy's bare. This was done so doctors would not confuse the two and would know which had been chosen to survive. Amy died two-thirds of the way through the five and a half hour surgery. Angela was stable after the procedure, but she died about ten months later, just before her first birthday.

Reitha Lakeberg seemed to dismiss the expense of the surgery, saying, "I can't live my life wondering if one of them, with that chance, would have lived." But others questioned whether a medical procedure should be performed when the costs are so high (hundreds of thousands of dollars, and the family had no medical insurance), the odds of survival are so low, and many people don't have access to basic health care because of a lack of funds.

Also, operations such as those done on the Lakeberg twins may violate the rule found in the Hippocratic Oath against a doctor hurting someone: "First, do no harm." Experts pointed out that if the twins had not been conjoined and they both were very ill, nobody would have suggested that one of them be sacrificed and her organs used to help the other survive. One said that society doesn't mind taking drastic measures with conjoined twins simply because people see them as monstrous.

But others see the separation of conjoined twins as a lifesaving procedure. When Christine and Betsy Wooden were born as conjoined twins in 1973, doctors separated them, and Betsy died of a heart defect. Christine is alive and well today. Their mother, Janna Walzeck, said, "They needed to be separated, and then what would happen, would happen. The stronger would survive, the weaker might not, but that was just—sometimes you have to sacrifice something to . . . get another life."

• CONJOINED TWINS ALIVE TODAY •

The Hensels, mentioned at the beginning of this chapter, are one pair of conjoined twins who remain united yet live normally.

They are *dicephalus* twins, and share—in addition to their one torso, two arms, and two legs—three lungs. The two each have a separate heart and stomach, but blood flows between

65

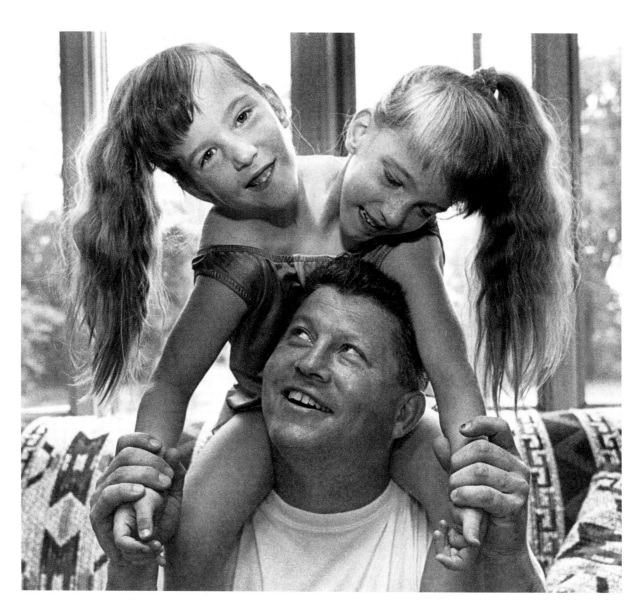

Abigail and Brittany with their dad. Abby is the right-side twin.

them. Their spines fuse at a single pelvis, and below the waist they share the organs that one person would have. Their condition is extremely rare. According to historical records, only four pairs of dicephalus twins have ever survived.

Each twin controls the arm and leg on her side. And each feels sensations just on her side, so when the twins get tickled on the left, only Britty giggles. But somehow they manage to coordinate their movements to walk, run, ride a bicycle, and swim. They have learned to sing and play piano together, with Abby playing the right-hand parts while her sister plays the left.

The children live in a small town in the Midwest, with their mother, an emergency-room nurse; their father, a carpenter/landscaper; and a younger brother and sister. They live on a farm with five cows, a horse, three dogs, and many cats. The people in their town treat them as normal, and when strangers are rude, they just ignore it. They point out to those who pry that they "don't have two heads" but in fact are two distinct people. Their clothing—purchased at stores, then modified by a seamstress to create two separate necklines—emphasizes this.

They have different tastes, personalities, and interests: Abby hates milk; Britty likes it. When they share soup, Britty insists that her sister not sprinkle the crackers on Britty's side. Abby likes to wear blue leggings, Britty prefers pink. Abby is the more aggressive twin, Britty the more artistic. Abby is better at math, while Britty is better at spelling.

The two make decisions by flipping a coin or taking turns, or their parents make a ruling. Usually they settle their differences by compromising, but not always. They've had arguments, and the occasional slap fight. Once, when they were very young, Britty hit Abby in the head with a rock.

Often, they seem to read each other's minds (one doctor thinks this may be because elements of their nervous systems overlap). When Britty coughs, Abby will automatically cover her sister's mouth with her hand. Once the two of them were watching TV when Abby said to Britty, "Are you thinking what I'm thinking?" Britty said yes, and they headed for their bedroom to read the same book.

Their parents tell them, "You can do anything." When they grow up, both want to be doctors. Britty says she also wants to get married and have children.

Another pair of conjoined twins who each have a good quality of life and a strong spirit are Lori and Dori (also known as Reba) Schappell. Born in Reading, Pennsylvania, in 1961, they are attached at the side of the head by parts of their skull and scalp, and by major blood vessels in their brains. Reba is paralyzed from the waist down, so Lori wheels her around in a special chair. These twins face in opposite directions, and maybe that's why they see life from different perspectives: Lori is outgoing, Reba is shy; Lori likes television, shopping, and sweets, Reba does not. Lori wears her brown hair short; Reba colors hers copper and has a wavy cut.

Both twins have pursued careers. Lori has worked as a clerk and a nurse-receptionist. Reba's passion is to be a country singer.

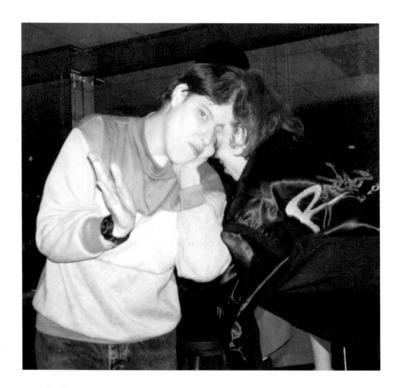

Lori (left) and Reba Schappell

conjoined
twins

She was recognized for special achievement at the Los Angeles Music Awards, which pays tribute to new artists. L.A. Music Awards founder Alfred Bowman said he was impressed with her talent and ability to perform under difficult circumstances.

The twins see themselves as being in many ways just like others. Reba says of their lives together, "There are good days and bad days—so what? This is what we know. We don't hate it. . . . I don't sit around questioning it or asking myself what I could do differently if I were separated."

The twins have developed effective ways of dealing with their needs for autonomy and privacy. They used to focus on Lori's career; now Lori works part time so Reba will have more time to develop her talents. When Reba sings at recording sessions or live performances, Lori becomes passive and lets her sister work. When Reba goes into her room, Lori doesn't talk.

On the other hand, Lori wants to get married and have babies. And when it comes to Lori's love life, it's Reba's turn to become quiet and let her mind drift off—so that while she's there physically, she's not really present. "The guy gets used to that," says Lori. "If he wants to be involved with me, he's got to get used to having her around."

Conjoined twins have much in common with other twins. They have an intense emotional bond—a bond made even closer by their physical connection. And like other twins, conjoined twins must resist being limited by this bond—they need to develop their own separate tastes and talents and become individuals. What sets conjoined twins apart are the physical challenges they confront and the prejudices of people who may see them as freakish. Their struggles to overcome these barriers make their stories some of the most compelling in the lives of twins.

• TWINS RESOURCES •

publications

Entwined Lives: Twins and What They Tell Us About Human Behavior, by Nancy L. Segal. New York: Dutton, 1999. A scientific look at twinship with many fascinating photographs.

Twins, photographs by David Fields, essays by Ruth and Rachel Sandweiss. Philadelphia: Running Press, 1998. Engaging portraits in words and photos of twenty-seven twin pairs.

Twins Magazine: Highly useful articles on health, psychology, and products for families with twins; photo essays too. Web site with sample articles from the current issue of the magazine, fun facts, resources, and links: www.twinsmagazine.com. Telephone: 1-888-55-TWINS. Address: 5350 S. Roslyn St., Suite 400, Englewood, CO 80111.

web sites

www.twinstuff.com: All the twinformation you could ever want, written by twins and for twins. Includes a photo gallery, essays, and twin diversions (including a twin screensaver, twin puzzle games, and a twin trivia quiz).

www.twinsfoundation.com: The Twins Foundation supports important research on twins. Their web site has articles, a gift shop where you can purchase books on twins, and links to other twin resources.

other

Twins Days Festival: Every year since 1976, twins and multiples from around the world have gathered in August in Twinsburg, Ohio (a town near Cleveland), to celebrate. For information, telephone 330-425-3652; log on to www.twinsdays.org; or e-mail info@twinsdays.org.

Twins Restaurant: Located in Manhattan in New York City, this restaurant is staffed exclusively by twins who work the same shift in the same stations while wearing the same uniform. Telephone: 1-800-RU-TWINS. E-mail: billywonka@aol.com. Web: www.twinsworld.com/restaurant.html

Casting Agency: If you have a double and want to be a star, contact Dreammakers, an agency run by the owners of the Twins Restaurant that places twins and multiples on TV shows, in advertising, and in movies. Address: Dreammakers, P.O. Box 6056, NY, NY 10128. Attn: Debbie and Lisa Ganz. Telephone: 1-800-RU-TWINS. Web: www.twinsworld.com/casting.html.

• SOURCE NOTES •

the world of twins

Lisa and Jennifer: personal interview.

HOW TWINS ARE MADE: "Multiple Birth," in *Encyclopedia Brittanica Online*; Randi Hutter Epstein, "You're Having Twins!" *Parents*, Aug. 1998, pp. 123–34; "Babies Born Weeks Apart," *New York Post*, September 18, 1980.

THE TWIN BOOM: National Center for Health Statistics, Centers for Disease Control and Prevention, "Births: Final Data for 1998," March 28, 2000; Epstein, p. 124.

THE MEANING OF "IDENTICAL": Nancy L. Segal, *Entwined Lives* (New York: Dutton, 1999), pp. 8-9, 28; CBS, *48 Hours*, July 8, 1999; Kenneth Ward, "Now I Know They're Fraternal," *Twins Magazine*, July/August 1995.

ANIMAL TWINS: Segal, pp. 230-38.

five dynamic duos

This chapter is based on personal interviews with the twins discussed and their families.

separated at birth

MY HEAD ON HIS SHOULDERS: CBS, *48 Hours*, July 8, 1999; Segal, pp. 111-12.

FRIENDS FOREVER: ABC, *20/20*, May 30, 1999; Carol Smith, "What It's Really Like to Be a Twin," *Redbook*, July 1998, p. 93; Nancy L. Segal, *Entwined Lives* (New York: Dutton, 1999), p. 2; Jill Neimark, Tracy Cochran, Larry Dossey, "Nature's Clones," *Psychology Today*, August 1997, pp. 36 ff.

THE ANGEL OF DEATH: Lucette Matalon Lagnado and Sheila Cohn Dekel, *Children of the Flames: Dr. Josef Mengele and the Untold Story of the Children of Auschwitz* (New York: William Morrow, 1991); Segal pp. 322-23.

THE GIGGLE TWINS: Segal, p. 127; Peter Watson, *Twins: An Uncanny Relationship* (New York: Viking, 1982), pp. 38-42; Neimark.

BIZARRE SIMILARITIES: Edwin Chen, "Twins Reared Apart," *New York Times Magazine*, Dec. 9, 1979, pp. 112 ff.

more amazing stories

WE THEE WED: Lucy Broadbent, "Twin Set," *Marie Claire*, Aug. 1997, pp. 40 ff; Ruth and Rachel Sandweiss, *Twins* (Philadelphia: Running Press, 1998), p. 60.

INCREDIBLE TWIN TEAMS: Sandweiss, pp. 32-37, 108.

READING MINDS: Kay Cassill, *Twins: Nature's Amazing Mystery* (New York: Atheneum, 1982), pp. 158-61.

THE SECRET LANGUAGE: Cassill, pp. 164-67; Flora Davis and Julia Orange, "The Twins Who Invented Their Own Language," *Redbook*, March 1978, pp. 113 ff.

THE DARK SIDE: Patrick McGrath, "The Death of the Silent Twin," *Harper's Bazaar*, Jan. 1, 1994, pp. 96ff. Jill Neimark, Tracy Cochran, Larry Dossey, "Nature's Clones," *Psychology Today*, August 1997, pp. 36 ff.

multiples

Quadruplets story: Panky Snow, "Quads Celebrating Birthdays," *Tampa Tribune*, Feb. 13, 1999, p. 18.

SEVENTH HEAVEN: Pam Belluck, "Iowan Makes U.S. History, Giving Birth to 7 Live Babies," *New York Times*, Nov. 20, 1997; Michael D. Lemonick, "'It's a Miracle,'" *Time*, Dec. 1, 1997, pp. 35 ff; Kathryn Casey, "See How They Grow," *Ladies Home Journal*, May 2000, pp. 167 ff.

MULTIPLE HAZARDS: Lance Morrow, "Is This Right?" *Time*, Jan. 11, 1999; Lemonick; Belluck; Kim Painter, "Risks and Costs Increase with Number of Fetuses," *USA Today*, November 10, 1997; "Encouraging Signs," ABCNEWS.com, Dec. 23, 1998.

AN IMPOSSIBLE CHOICE: Maureen West, "Fertility Treatments Force Parents with Too Many Fetuses to Make Life or Death Choices," *Arizona Republic*, Feb. 21, 1999.

THE BIG SHOW: Lemonick, p. 39; Sylvia Chase, Diane Sawyer, Sam Donaldson, "Once Upon a Time," *ABC Primetime Live*, November 26, 1997; Barry Came, "A Family Tragedy," *Maclean's*, Nov. 21, 1994, pp. 40 ff.

conjoined twins

UNITED FROM BIRTH and THE HISTORICAL RECORD: Laura E. Beardsley, "Body Doubles: Siamese Twins in Fact and Fiction" (notes to an exhibition at the Mutter Museum in Philadelphia), 1995; "Conjoined Twin," in *Encyclopedia Brittanica Online*; Nancy L. Segal, *Entwined Lives* (New York: Dutton, 1999), pp. 295-312.

THE DILEMMA OF SEPARATION: Segal, p. 306; Anastasia Toufexis, "Medicine: The Ultimate Choice," *Time*, Aug. 30, 1993, p. 43; Natalie Angier/New York Times News Service, "Twins Conjoined at the Head Living Life to the Fullest," *Dallas Morning News*, Jan. 4, 1998; Nancy Snyderman and Diane Sawyer, "Two Lives," *ABC Primetime Live*, March 11, 1998.

CONJOINED TWINS ALIVE TODAY: Kenneth Miller, "Together Forever," *Life*, April 1, 1996; Claudia Wallis, "Medicine: The Most Intimate Bond," *Time*, March 25, 1996, pp. 60 ff; Kenneth Miller, "Conjoined Twins Abby and Britty Hensel Present Their World," *Life*, Sept. 1, 1998, pp. 34 ff; Ruth and Rachel Sandweiss, *Twins* (Philadelphia: Running Press, 1998), pp. 124-29; Angier.

71

• INDEX •

Illustrations appear in italic

a

animal twins and multiples, 9

b

birth defects, 13, 19, 45, 48, 50

bond between twins, 16–17, 21, 35, 36, 41

Botsch, Martha, 28–29

Bunker, Chang and Eng, 58–60, *59*

c

cesarean sections, 12, 46

Chukwu octuplets, 49–50, *49*

Chulkhurst, Mary and Eliza, 57–58, *58*

circuses, 58, 60, 63

community support, 46, 50

concentration camps, 30, 31

conception, 2; fertility treatments and, 5, 44, 45

conjoined twins, 5, 55–69; exploitation of, 60–61, 63; historical explanations of, 57; marriage and, 60, 62, 63, 69; performances by, 58, 61–62, 63, 69; surgery to separate, 60, 64–65

Curry, Stephanie, 28–29

Curry-Wills quadruplets, 43–44, *44*

d

dating, 16, 20–21, 35

difficulties raising multiples, 12–13, 43, 48

Dionne quintuplets, 43, *43*, 51–54, *52*, *53*

display and exploitation, 51, 52–53, 60–61, 63; *see also* conjoined twins, exploitation of

DNA tests, 7

e

Entwined Lives, 60

ethical conflicts, 48, 50, 65

expenses, 48, 50

extrasensory perception, 38–39, 67

f

fertility treatments 5–6, 44, 51

fraternal twins, 2, 3

Freaks, 63

g

genes, 3, 6, 28, 33, 55; genetic traits, 28, 30, 32, 33

Gibbons, June and Jennifer, 40–41

Goodship, Daphne, 32, *32–33*

Gould, Jennifer and Lisa, *viii*, 1, *1*, 16–18, *17*, *18*

Greenfield, Max and Andy, 13–16, *14*, *15*

h

Han, Gina and Sunny, 41–42

Hensel, Abigail and Brittany, 55, *55*, 65–68, *66*

Herbert, Barbara, 32, *32–33*

heredity; *see* genes; nature-vs.-nurture

Hilton, Violet and Daisy, 62–64, *63*

Hollenbeck, Scott and Sean, 36–38, *37*

i

identical twins, 2, 3, 6–9, 23, 55

in-vitro fertilization, 45, 51

k

Kennedy, Gracie and Ginny, 39–40

l

Lakeberg, Amy and Angela, 64–65

languages, private, 39, 40

Lassen, Jena and Jill, *34*, 34–35

Levey, Jerry, *26*, 26–27

Lewis, Jim, 33

m

Malm, Phil and Doug, *34*, 34–35

marriage, 17–18, 34–36, 60, 62, 63

Martin, Kathy and Arleen, 19–21, *19*, *20*

McCaughey septuplets, 45–46, *47*, 50, 54

McGregor Cal and Ali, *35*, 35–36

Mendez, Robert and Ralph, 38

Mengele, Dr. Josef, 30–31

Messina, Andrea and children, *10*, 10–13, *11*, *12*

Millie-Christine, *61*, 61–62

Moriarty, Erin and Sheelah, 6–7, *7*

Mozes, Eva, 30

multiple births, 43–54; causes of, 2–3, 4–5, 55–56, 57; dangers, 48; increases in, 5, 44

n

nature-vs.-nurture, 27–28, 33

Nazi Germany, 30–31

Newman, Mark, 26, 27

o

octuplets, 49

p

parasitic twins, 56–57

Partridge, Ron and Pad, 21–25, *22*, *25*

Plompen, Terri, 4

Poto and Cabengo, 39–40

pregnancy, 10–11, 12, 19, 46, 48, 49; risks of, 45, 48, 49, 51; competition in womb, 4, 6

premature birth, 12, 46, 48

q

quadruplets, 43–44

quintuplets, 43, 51–54

r

relationship between twins, 16–18, 20–21, 35, 38, 40–42

s

Schappell, Lori and Reba (Dori), 68, 68–69

Seemuth, Kelley and Missi, 6

Segal, Nancy, 60

selective termination, 45, 49, 50–51

separation of twins, 17, 28–29, 40–41

septuplets, 45–46, 50, 54

Siamese twins, 58; *see also* conjoined twins

sonograms, 4, *4*

Springer, Jim, 33

Stanch, Jim and Jeff, *35*, 35–36

statistics, 3, 5, 44, 56

supertwins, 5; *see also* multiple births

surgery, 64, 65

t

Tedesco, Jimmy, 26–27

time span between births, 4

Tocci, Giacomo and Giovanni, 62, *62*

Twins Day Festival, 34, 35

Twinsburg, Ohio, 34

w

wheelchair racing, 37–38

Wooden, Christine and Betsy, 65